What people say al

"I didn't have masses to lose, but was tired of feeling bloated around my middle, and carrying a bit too much extra fat all over my body. My aim was to feel a little leaner, and to re-set my eating habits after a winter of comfort food and sugar laden treats.

The Nitro+ Diet was easy to understand, and very simple to follow. I'd lost 8 pounds in the first 4 weeks (my target was 10) and my measurements showed losses in all of my target zones. Scrambled eggs have become my all-time favourite breakfast, and I have built protein into my regular eating habits, meaning I don't snack as much and am eating far less sugar.

My weight is now steady at my target, and I feel really confident that I will be able to maintain it with my re-educated approach to eating.

However, should Christmas, or a holiday excesses take their toll I will return to the diet as a kick start to get back to the weight I am happiest at." – *Jill Willis*

The
Nitro+ Diet

James Murray

Rapid, lasting fat reduction
Ignite your muscles in just four weeks

Published by Magic Pocket 2017
ISBN: 978-1530554256

Design and layout by Hafiz Ladell
for Magic Pocket Productions
www.magicpocket.co.uk

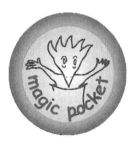

Table of Contents

Acknowledgements

There are many people I would like to thank. My wife Nicola who has put up with me for nearly 20 years . . . I couldn't have done it without her. My lovely mum, who I lost to cancer in 2014, who gave me so much drive, belief and inspiration . . . I miss her every day. To my Dad for his encouragement and to my children Abigail, Elliot and Jensen, whom I am extremely proud of – you make me smile every day.

   I would like to thank Jo Adshead for her help in editing and proofreading, my friend and squash partner Dr Kirk Graham for kindly writing my foreword, and not forgetting my very patient editor Hafiz, who has been fantastic in pulling all this together and getting a book out of me. ☺

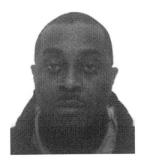

Foreword
by
Dr Kirk Graham MBBS

**Emergency Medicine Specialist
PGDip (Diabetes)**

The UK is seen to have the highest level of obesity in Western Europe, ahead of countries such as France, Germany, Spain and Sweden. Levels of obesity in the UK have more than trebled in the last 30 years. It is currently estimated that more than half the population could be obese by 2050.

According to the UN Food and Agriculture Organisation one in four British adults is obese, which has led to fears that the UK has become the "fat man of Europe".

Obesity can lead to several other serious life threatening illnesses such as diabetes and hypertension which, combined, will cost the UK billions of pounds in prevention, education and treatment over the coming years. An epidemic of gigantic proportions is waiting to happen.

With this in mind the UK needs an urgent solution. This book will provide a guide to nutrition, fitness and exercise. Following the simple principles set down in these pages will make you healthier, fitter, slimmer and happier.

James Murray is a fitness enthusiast, keen squash player and fitness entrepreneur. He is always interested in improving the health and wellbeing of other persons.

For my family

Introduction

Are you ready to change your life? Read this book and find out how transformation is possible: increase your energy levels, boost your fitness, change your body shape, restore your confidence and self esteem . . . And, perhaps best of all, you'll learn how to banish unwanted body fat forever.

Maybe this all sounds like a tall order, but you'll discover that it's not as hard as you might think to change your shape and burn off body fat – you just need to make sure certain principles are in place. This book is going to tell you what these principles are. Remember these principles, post them on your fridge, tattoo them on your hand, email them to yourself . . . the important thing is to remember them, and to put them into practice. They will serve you well, long after you've scrubbed off that tattoo!

The Nitro+ Diet has been developed over many years of paying attention to what works. It's all about being smart when it comes to diet and exercise. So, how smart are you?

When people join a gym it's normally for the same reason – to lose fat, lean out and get fitter. You may have noticed how gym membership goes through the roof after Christmas, and then again midway through the year when the holiday season approaches. It drives me mad – people are hanging around the gym like the smell of old socks. But that's what people are like. Either they are feeling guilty about all those mince pies they couldn't say no to, or they are anxious about the kind of figure they're going to cut on the beach. There's a sudden frenzy of crash diets and personal trainers, fuelled by the urge to change moobs into pecs and muffin tops into bikini bods. If we reckon we look good, we feel good.

Give yourself a break, people!

I've designed some new gym products that can be used at home or in the gym. Believe me, they are great.

The Bellmate Kinetic is a multi-purpose conditioning and fitness apparatus that can also turn into a muscle release or massage tool. It can be used in the gym, at home or on your travels. It's an amazing piece of kit, allowing the user to complete well over a hundred exercises – now that is smart.

And there's the new Bellmate Evolve, the only aerobic stepper that can transform into a fully functional workout bench, supporting dumbbells, barbells and resistance bands, as well as allowing users to do over one hundred exercises on just one piece of equipment.

The Nitro+ Diet will get you where you want to go faster and more effectively than any other diet out there. Practise the 5 step MAXIM method and your body will be changing in front of your eyes. Fat will be falling off you! You'll become part of the new, exciting Kinetic revolution that is going to change the fitness industry forever.

Take a look at our website *www.bellmatesystems.com* for FREE calculators, blogs and FREE one month access to the complete Kinetic Fit System. Just get your unique code on page 274 and enter it on our website.

What is the Nitro+ Diet?

Over the past 30 years there have been literally hundreds of new diets and programmes, all promising to help you lose weight, strip body fat, drop a dress size etc, etc. In your local bookstore, or when you look online, there are so many diet books to choose from, but how are you going to know what really works? So many different angles: counting calories, partitioning foods, eating raw, cutting out carbohydrates, eating more protein, eating more fat, eating sprouts, eating figs, eating celery, fasting, fruiting . . . to name just a few. It's a fat loss minefield, a zone of confusion bordering on despair.

So, what is the Nitro+ Diet? It sounds like something out of a monster truck show! But don't worry, I won't be advising you to tuck into liquid nitrogen . . . that would be just plain silly, wouldn't it? I do still have fond memories from my school Science classes, where my teacher, Mr Carpenter, would pass round a jar of liquid nitrogen, instructing us all on no account to touch or dabble our fingers in it. That's like asking kids not to lick the cake bowl – of course that's exactly what they'll do. I just hope those kids didn't have lunch straight afterwards!

No, I'm with Mr Carpenter on this: definitely don't try eating it. So, what's with the zany title?

Nitro+ is fast, punchy, explosive and delivers rapid results – think nitroglycerin! It's also short for Nitrogen. We'll be finding out a lot about Nitrogen, what it does in your body, and how it can help burn off your body fat. It'll be a fascinating exploration of the highways and byways of the human metabolism, but best of all, it'll provide you with a route map to get to the place you want to be.

What makes this system different?

Reading this book will change your life. It contains very important principles that you can easily remember and will educate you on how to create the best fat burning environment.

It's not just about a diet, either; there's an integrated exercise system, described in detail in Step 4–Ignite. I've developed the most effective anabolic exercises, which, in combination with the Bellmate Kinetic, can cause your muscles to ignite into fat burning furnaces. Performing these exercises three times a week is just as important as following the Nitro+ Diet. They'll work together syner-getically, creating the conditions that will burn off all that godforsaken fat. Your muscles will ignite into an anabolic powerhouse, switching on your internal system for trans-forming stored fats into energy.

If you don't do much exercise and consume lots of car-bohydrates and fats your muscles never experience the call for nutritional fuel, so fat builds up very easily. Your fat burning mechanism is turned off; you forgot where the switch is! Maybe you're thinking, exercise is just going to make me tired . . . but the amazing truth is, exercise will energise!

You know those times when you've left your a car in a long stay airport car park? When you come back the damn thing just isn't going to start; the battery's flat – never mind va-va-voom, there's not even a single ounce of oomph. The body acts the same way; without regular exercise it simply doesn't get to recharge. You end up feeling just like a sad sack, without even the energy to shift off the sofa.

Follow the methods and stick to the principles in this book and I guarantee it will switch on your muscle messengers and turn off the fat storage mechanism. It'll be your first step to greatness. Like the Nike slogan says – JUST DO IT.

Nitrogen
is everywhere!

What is nitrogen? Where is it found? How can it help me get lean?

You see, Mr Carpenter, I was paying attention in your science lessons – unlike those idiots who were busy scoffing down the liquid nitrogen!

Nitrogen is literally everywhere. It's one of the most common elements in the universe, round about seventh in terms of abundance in the Milky Way and the Solar System. Here on Mother Earth it comprises about 78% of our atmosphere – i.e. most of the air that you breathe.

In the periodic table of chemical elements its symbol is N, with the atomic number 7. We can visualise its atomic structure as a central core of seven protons and neutrons, surrounded by two concentric rings of electrons – just like on the cover of this book!

Diet and the human body

The human body contains about 3% by mass of nitrogen, which is the fourth most abundant element in the body after oxygen, carbon, and hydrogen. It's an important part of our food intake, a crucial constituent of the amino and nucleic acids vital for our survival.

Nitrogen is abundant in protein foods and also occurs in substances called purines, which play an important role in the body's metabolic process. These purines are present in many different foods and also occur naturally in the body.

I'll be showing you how in today's world we don't eat enough nitrogen rich foods – and when we do eat them, we do so at the wrong times.

Protein

Protein is very important: the human body requires it for both growth and maintenance. Aside from water, proteins are the most abundant kind of molecules in the body. It is the major structural component of all cells, particularly muscle cells. Body organs, hair and skin: all rely on protein.

Glycoproteins in membranes play an important role in cell-to-cell interactions. When broken down into amino acids, proteins are useful as precursors to nucleic acids, co-enzymes, hormones, immune response, cellular repair, and the production of other molecules essential for life. Additionally, protein is needed to form blood cells.

Every 100 grams of protein contains around 16 grams of nitrogen, i.e. 16%.

High protein foods that are rich in nitrogen include:

Meat and Poultry

The mainstays of our Western diet – beef, pork, lamb, chicken and turkey – are all important sources of protein. In particular, the organ meats (such as liver, kidney, tripe, heart, even brain) of these animals contain high amounts of protein and purines. The healthiest cuts are those with the least saturated fats – the stuff that makes you fat, loads up the saddle bags and spreads icing all over your muffin tops.

I would recommend eating more fish, poultry and high protein vegetables and limiting red meat to just once a week.

Fish and Seafood

These are my favourite high protein foods. Not only are they are packed with nitrogen, courtesy of their high purine and protein content, they also have plenty of omega-3 fish oils, so beneficial for heart health and so helpful in losing body fat. Seafoods high in omega-3 include herring, salmon, mackerel and sardines. Other fish combining very high protein with low fat include cod, halibut, and tuna.

When selecting tuna, go for the light chunks or skip-jack, as this tends to be lower in mercury than other tuna. Why should we worry about mercury? Nearly all fish and shellfish contain traces of mercury, but the risk is minimal for most people and is not normally a health concern. Nonetheless, the higher levels of mercury present in some fish may be harmful to pregnant women, and you'll want to be particularly careful what fish you give to your kids, since too much mercury can damage their growing nervous systems. It's best to avoid king mackerel, tilefish, swordfish and shark, all likely to have high mercury levels. Instead, stick to low mercury seafood such as shrimp, salmon, pollock, skipjack tuna and catfish.

Here's a guide identifying four groups, to help you make your choice. My advice: stick to the first two groups and steer clear of the last two groups (High and Highest).

Guide to safe levels of mercury in fish

Least mercury: *feel free to enjoy these fish*

Anchovies	Butterfish	Catfish
Clam	Crab	Crayfish
Croaker (Atlantic)	Flounder	Hake
Haddock (Atlantic)	Herring	Mackerel
Chub	Mullet	Oyster
Perch (Ocean)	Plaice	Pollock
Salmon (fresh)	Salmon (canned)	Sardine
Scallop	Shad (American)	Shrimp
Sole (Pacific)	Squid (Calamari)	Tilapia
Trout (Freshwater)	Whitefish	Whiting

Moderate mercury: *max 6 servings/month*

Bass (Striped, Black)	Carp	Cod (Alaskan)
Croaker (White Pacific)	Halibut (Atlantic)	Lobster
Jacksmelt (Silverside)	Halibut (Pacific)	Mahi Mahi
Tuna (Skipjack)	Perch (Freshwater)	Monkfish
Tuna (canned light)	Sablefish	Snapper
Weakfish (Sea Trout)	Skate	

High mercury: *max 3 servings/month*

Mackerel (Spanish, Gulf)	Sea Bass (Chilean)
Canned Albacore Tuna	Tuna (Yellowfin)
Bluefish	Grouper

Highest mercury: *avoid these completely*

Mackerel (King)	Orange Roughy	Marlin
Shark	Swordfish	Tilefish
Tuna (Big eye, Ahi)		

Fruit and Vegetables

Legumes (peas, beans, lentils) and soya products are the only types of vegetables that are high in protein. However, some fruits and vegetables are high in purines and will therefore contribute to your nitrogen intake. Apart from legumes, these include cauliflower, spinach, green peas and asparagus.

Green leafy vegetables can be nutritional power-houses. When Popeye gets into a tight spot, he won't be calling for a plate of bacon and eggs; instead, a quick tin of spinach emptied down his gullet sets his biceps instantly a-quiver. Me too, I love spinach – it's a vegetable dynamo. It's best eaten raw, to take advantage of the high levels of potassium (good for blood pressure) and the vitamins A and C that bolster and strengthen our immune system. And that's not all: spinach is also high in protein and bursting with folates, calcium, magnesium and manganese, all minerals vital for healthy bones, high energy levels and cell growth and maintenance.

Fruits are full of vitamins, minerals and fibre but are not naturally high in protein or purines. Some fruits, however, are worth special consideration. In Step 3 – eXchange I'll tell you about some of my favourite fruits which do contain significant amounts of protein.

Berries belong in a special class of superfruit, being particularly loaded with vitamins and minerals. Blueberries, blackberries and cranberries are great for your immune system and general health.

Other Foods

Dairy products, eggs, nuts and seeds all provide protein, and therefore nitrogen, although they're low-purine foods. Whole grains, including wheat and oats, also provide some purines and protein.

I recommend choosing low fat dairy products, watching your serving sizes of nuts and seeds (owing to their high fat content) and limiting eggs to no more than four per week, owing to their high cholesterol content. Now, I often have more than four eggs in a week but by removing some of the yolks before scrambling I'm able to keep the cholesterol under control. And in place of milk, why not try soya milk? I drink it all the time – it's high in protein and, unlike normal cows' milk, low in carbohydrates, plus the taste is actually quite good.

Maintaining a positive nitrogen balance

This is very important; it's what this diet centres around. By following the five step MAXIM methods and sticking to the Nitro+ Principles you will switch your body from a negative nitrogen balance to a healthy positive nitrogen balance (PNB). This positive state is where the nitrogen intake is greater than the nitrogen output.

When we are in a PNB our muscles are much more receptive to nutrients and less likely to collapse. The vast majority of overweight or obese people are in a catabolic state and a negative nitrogen balance. Their muscles are simply not switched on, and therefore not burning energy as effectively as they could. It's like a steam train with no one available to shovel coal into the furnaces (not that I'm an old-timer, but you must have seen this set-up in the old Western movies).

Through eating the right foods and following a good exercise routine, muscles are switched on and become receptive to nutrients. Most people have the idea that leaner people have a higher basal metabolic rate and overweight people slower metabolic rates. Actually, the word metabolism refers to how much energy your body uses, or how many calories you burn in a day. This means that the heavier you are the higher your basal metabolic rate is going to be, in consequence of your carrying additional weight, and vice versa.

Looks can, however, be deceiving. Low calorie diets have been popular for the past two decades, especially with models. Some supermodels have a reported body fat of over 30% – amazingly, these supermodels are borderline obese! They may look healthy from the outside, but on the inside they are in a permanent catabolic negative nitrogen state and are literally wasting away. Retaining muscle tissue is ESSENTIAL to losing body fat. Think of muscle tissue as the steam engine furnace where body fat is burned. Building stronger muscles will lead to improved posture, muscle tone, joints and general health. Moreover, lean muscle that is toned and active will burn body fat even when you are sleeping.

Switch on your muscles, turn on your fat burners and ignite your engine. What's stopping you? Believe in yourself – you are great and you can achieve anything.

RDAs for protein are a load of cobblers

Recommended daily amounts, especially for protein, are nonsense. That's right, they make no sense at all; they're gobbledegook.

We are always being encouraged to eat plenty of carbohydrates, even though when the liver and muscle storage is full, the carbohydrate will be stored as body fat. With regard to protein, in the UK the RDA for women aged between 19 and 70 years old is a paltry 46 grams per day (based on a 57.5 kg individual). For men aged between 19 and 70 RDA is also very low: 56 grams of protein per day (based on a 70 kg individual). These recommended daily quantities of protein – equating to roughly 0.8 grams of protein per kilogram of bodyweight – are based on a normal sedentary lifestyle. True, if you are more active then a higher RDA of carbohydrate is suggested; I agree that this is necessary in order to access readily available energy from stored glycogen, but the RDAs for protein are still way too low.

An interesting experiment

A study was conducted in 2013 by the Human Use Review Committee at the U.S. Army Research Institute of Environmental Medicine and the Institutional Review Board at the University of North Dakota.

The resulting paper was titled "Effects of high-protein diets on fat-free mass and muscle protein synthesis following weight loss: a randomized controlled study". Its purpose was to determine the effects of varying levels of dietary protein on body composition and muscle protein synthesis when dieting or in energy deficit ('ED').

The trial involved 39 adults, divided into three groups according to their prescribed protein intake as follows:

Protein Levels	
Group 1	RDA @ 0.8 grams per Kg
Group 2	RDA x 2, i.e.1.6 grams per Kg
Group 3	RDA x 3, i.e 2.4 grams per Kg

The study lasted for 31 days. For the first 10 days the volunteers were all on a normal weight management diet, following which the three different levels of protein intake were imposed. At the same time everyone's calories were reduced by approximately 30% while the level of exercise was increased by 10%, resulting in a 40% energy deficit over days 11–31.

Given that reducing calories is known to reduce body weight, the purpose of this experiment was to determine how protein levels can affect fat free mass (muscle) and fat mass when dieting or reducing calorie intake. The study concluded that, although health related outcomes are often improved with the loss of body weight owing to decline in body fat, as much as 25% of total body loss may comprise skeletal muscle mass. In overweight and obese individuals, reductions in muscle mass may restrict further weight loss and compromise weight management regimes by impeding normal metabolic processes, including protein turnover and basal metabolic rate.

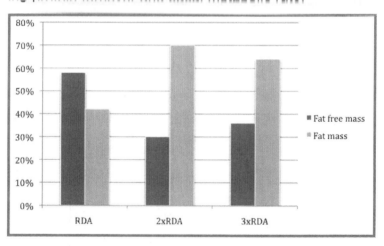

Here's a graph neatly summarising what happened to the various groups during the final three weeks of the experiment (days 11 to 31). All three groups lost body weight in this time, but there was a clear difference in the proportions of fat to muscle constituting the lost body mass.

The greatest loss of weight occurred amongst the RDAx1 group: around 3.6 kgs (7.92 lbs), of which 58% was fat free mass (muscle) and 42% was body fat. Amongst the RDAx2 group not so much overall weight was lost (2.5 Kg / 5.5lb in total), but this included a significantly higher percentage – 28% more – of body fat than Group 1. This amounts to just under half a pound more fat loss than the RDA group. Results for the RDAx3 group were also very impressive: there was a total loss of around 3 kgs (6.6 lbs), comprising 36% muscle loss and 64% vanished fat.

The study also measured the nitrogen levels in each group from day 9 to day 30, registering a fall at day 11, when the calories were reduced, for all participants. For the remainder of the study Group 1 remained negative; nitrogen levels for Group 3 showed a gradual increase without ever returning to a positive balance; whilst only Group 2 succeeded in returning to a positive state, achieving this by day 17.

These results clearly demonstrate the advantages of eating more protein in your diet when calories have been reduced. In my opinion the protein intake of the RDAx3 group was excessive; the Nitro+ Diet bears most resemblance to the RDAx2 group. In this group not only was weight loss slower and more gradual, but more fat was burned and the least amount of muscle lost.

This is significant, because muscle retention is the key to fat-burning success. **The more lean muscle tissue you have, the more calories you will burn.**

As the study shows, the RDAx2 regime offered the most effective levels of protein for burning body fat and maintaining a positive nitrogen balance. The Nitro+ Diet recommends very similar protein intake levels, which will burn off 30% more fat than the so-called recommended daily intake regime.

It's a very important conclusion to draw; do feel free to read carefully through this section again so you can take it in properly. It proves that protein in the right amounts can create a positive nitrogen balance and burn body fat more efficiently than anything else – and that's for definite.

Obesity – a global crisis

It's not just the UK that's getting fatter – it's happening all over the world. It's a serious problem that's in danger of running out of control, like a snowball gaining in size and momentum as it rolls down the hill. Watch out! – eventually it could flatten us all.

According to the World Health Organisation (WHO) at least 2.8 million people are dying each year as a result of being overweight or obese. In the UK an astonishing 64% of adults – that's nearly two thirds of the adult population – are overweight, according to data from Public Health England. In Europe, only Hungary has a higher percentage of obesity. We need to act now to stop this march of the muffin tops, moobs and saddle bags.

Studies into obesity prevention have indicated that giving up watching television for a week reduces a child's waist size by an average 2.3 cm (just under an inch). In 2008, over 40 million preschool children worldwide were overweight! So rather than plonking your kids in front of the TV, computer or tablet, get them outside on their bikes or playing sport, like we did when you and I were kids. There I go again, talking like an old-timer! Back in the day we hardly watched any TV. Not that there was much worth watching – but I do remember the A team, Neighbours and Eastenders . . . Still, I'd rather have been out playing football, skateboarding, rollerblading, playing rounders, climbing trees, playing knock down ginger . . . all those physical things. Just think about how our kids are going to look and feel when they get older. We as parents can do something about this now – don't leave it till it's too late. You can start by reducing the amount of fruit juice and fizzy drinks they guzzle down. Try to get them to eat some breakfast, and hide away the sweets and crisps. Don't put it off, do it now – however much they might moan now, your kids will thank you later . . . before they are 30 and after they've waved goodbye to those challenging teenage years.

Our waists are expanding along with our portion sizes, and that can't be good news. In the UK it's costing the NHS billions of pounds. An analysis of data from 1980 to 2013 indicates that British people have over this time become ever more overweight or obese, so that the UK is now third in the shameful European league table of excess weight, just behind Iceland and Malta. It's gone way beyond a joke – it's a bloody problem, a huge problem.

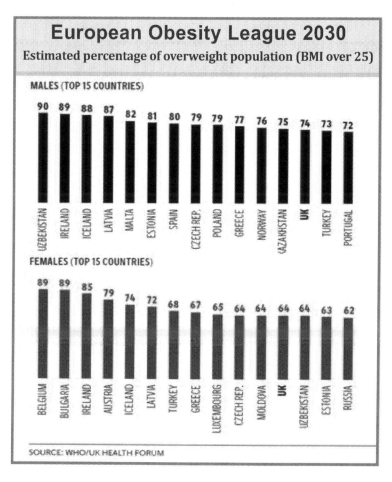

European Obesity League 2030
Estimated percentage of overweight population (BMI over 25)

MALES (TOP 15 COUNTRIES)

90 UZBEKISTAN, 89 IRELAND, 88 ICELAND, 87 LATVIA, 82 MALTA, 81 ESTONIA, 80 SPAIN, 79 CZECH REP., 79 POLAND, 77 GREECE, 76 NORWAY, 75 KAZAKHSTAN, 74 UK, 73 TURKEY, 72 PORTUGAL

FEMALES (TOP 15 COUNTRIES)

89 BELGIUM, 89 BULGARIA, 85 IRELAND, 79 AUSTRIA, 74 ICELAND, 72 LATVIA, 68 TURKEY, 67 GREECE, 65 LUXEMBOURG, 64 CZECH REP., 64 MOLDOVA, 64 UK, 64 UZBEKISTAN, 63 ESTONIA, 62 RUSSIA

SOURCE: WHO/UK HEALTH FORUM

The study defines being overweight as having a Body Mass Index (BMI) of 25 or more, with scores of over 30 counting as obese. In the UK, well over half the adult population – 67% of men and 57% of women – fall into these two categories. BMI may no longer be the cutting edge metric, but it does allow us to get a handle on the scale of the problem. It demands an effective response, one that will result in us not only looking better, but also feeling more energised, and bursting with renewed self esteem and confidence.

Even more shocking are the figures for children and adolescents. The study found 26% of boys and 29% of girls were overweight or obese, compared to 17.5% and 21% in 1980. These statistics are disturbing, to say the least. My idea of adolescence involves kids running around, screaming their heads off, fuelled by an apparently inexhaustible supply of energy; but instead, kids are just getting fatter, more bloated, glued to the sofa.

So what's been going on? I'm going to spread the blame here – on the supermarkets and fast food restaurants, but also on parents.

Fast food is advertised like it's a whole fun, empowering way of life, but really it's all about money. Who do you think are two of the largest sponsors for the up and coming 2016 Olympics and the 2018 World Cup? Yep, no prizes for guessing – Coca Cola and McDonalds.

We've fallen in love with the American fast food lifestyle, without pausing to consider the consequences. There are more McDonalds, KFC, Burger King, Pizza Hut, Pizza Xpress restaurants popping up on our high streets every week. They're offering cheap, convenient food high in simple refined carbohydrates, saturated fats and salt, all sloshed down with half a litre of sugary flavoured water. Kids love it – but it's full of crap. Hey, parents, I have some important advice: it's time to stop feeding your kids this rubbish.

Most obese and overweight people are permanently in

a catabolic, negative nitrogen state. Their metabolism is simply not configured towards burning body fat – their fat burning engines remain dormant. The Nitro+ Diet is different: it engages with scientific principle to turn off the catabolic process and switch on the fat burner. Catabolic means muscle wasting; it's what happens when you follow traditional low fat, low carbohydrate diets.

The illustration below compares statistics for obesity from 1993 and 2012. In just 19 years obesity levels expanded by 11.2% for males and 8.7% for females. The graph across the page tracks the increase over this period more precisely.

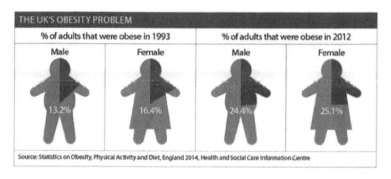

Analysis of trend data from 188 countries worldwide shows that the proportion of male adults with a BMI of 25 or more increased from 29% in 1980 to 37% in 2013, while for female adults there was a rise from 30% to 38% over the same period.

Things are looking particularly bad in the States, where almost 70% of Americans are overweight. Now, I've been lucky enough to spend time in the USA, and I love the American people – they are delightful, very friendly and

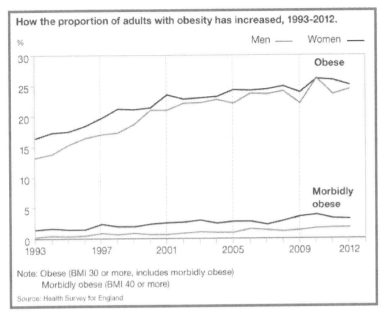

How the proportion of adults with obesity has increased, 1993-2012.

Men —— Women ——

Obese

Morbidly obese

Note: Obese (BMI 30 or more, includes morbidly obese)
Morbidly obese (BMI 40 or more)
Source: Health Survey for England

always helpful. But they just eat too darn much – and it's not that they're being consciously greedy. The portion sizes are ridiculous. Go into any restaurant and ask for something large and it will come out on a wheelbarrow! Ask for a large drink and you get a bucket, ask for a coffee and the waitress comes over five more times to check if you want a refill. I remember one trip to a pizza pie restaurant where the customers looked a match for the serving sizes. Me, I could only manage one slice and took the other slices home – they lasted me a whole week!

New predictions from the World Health Organization suggest that three in every four men and two in every three women will be overweight by 2030. Read that again, slowly . . . take it on board. It's looking particularly serious in Ireland, on course for an obesity epidemic: researchers predict that by 2030 36% of men and 30% of women will have a BMI higher than 30.

The consequences are likely to be dire: hospitals are going to be filled with overweight people seeking treatment for associated problems such as type 2 diabetes, heart and lung malfunctions, fatty liver, arthritis, poor joint function and weak bones and muscles. But still we act as if nothing is happening! Our supermarket shelves continue to be stacked high with tempting offers of refined high fat, high sugar convenience foods. On every high street the fast food chains make it as easy as pie to load up on junk, because that's what we seem to like. It's high time to wise up – if we carry on like this we're all going to end up in hospital, surrendering years off our natural lifespan.

This obesity crisis is enormous. We need to take action – now.

Supermarkets, profits and obesity

Uh-oh, I seem to have got my finger jammed on the rant button. Don't worry, I'm not going to spend too long on this one – I could easily write another book on the links between supermarkets, fast food restaurants and obesity, but that'll have to wait for another day. The simple truth is that both the supermarkets and the fast food restaurants are a major factor in why we continue to get fatter.

Our love affair with new technology is also playing its part. These days virtually everyone keeps a smart phone, tablet or whizzy tech device within grasping distance. We feel the need to be permanently connected to the internet, email, messages, social media, etc, just in case we might miss something on the crazy interactive virtual universe that forms our new social reality. How many times have I walked into a café and seen the majority of customers hunkered down over their little screens, busy with who knows what . . . whilst sitting down? So many hours a day wrapped up in careless postures, oblivious to what's going on just across the table, chasing the next distraction. Fact is, apps like facebook, twitter and instagram are designed to waste your time (and maybe that's why we love them!). I see people all the time in the gym checking their facebook and twitter updates. It's the knowledge equivalent of junk food – chowing down on meaningless trivia under the pretence of staying connected and informed.

Convenience foods – mostly salty, crunchy, fatty parcels of carbohydrate – are the perfect partner to an hour or three hunched over a screen. You dip your hand in the bag from time to time, crunch and swallow . . . crunch and swallow . . . before you know it it's time to order another bag. No wonder supermarket shelves are loaded down with this stuff.

There's a lot of thought and calculation that goes into supermarket design. When you walk through the doors you feel welcomed by the delicious aroma of freshly-baked bread, cheered by the delightful flower displays. Everything is abundant, and all of it could be yours! Cheery music plays soft and gentle in the background. Your heart rate slows, you feel calm and relaxed. But don't be fooled – it's just the supermarkets getting you in the mood to spend your hard earned cash. And, most likely, you'll end up spending loads more than you'd planned.

The special deals – three for the price of two, buy one get one free (BOGOF!), are always for the junkiest stuff, unhealthy, high sugar, fat, salt foods. Go on – it's almost like we're giving it away. Sometimes it is being given away: staff members blocking the aisle, pressing free samples of chocolate, crisps, cheesy snacks, even plastic beakers of wine into your hand, and all with the cynical understanding that, having accepted something for free, you'll feel some sort of obligation to load a whole lot more of it into your trolley. And bear in mind, research has shown that if you double the size of your trolley, you'll buy 40% more items.

Of course, there's a lot more filling the supermarket shelves than just plain junk. We all need to eat, and it is possible to eat extremely well from supermarket produce. You just need to pay a little more attention while you shop. Instead of simply grabbing a pre-packed bag of veggies, take your time to make your own selection. Hunt out the real bargains on the higher and lower shelves, and take the trouble to track down the staple goods so unhelpfully stocked in the further corners of the shop. Most important of all, resist the urge to take the easy route down junkfood alley. Be especially alert as you head towards the check-out, past the rows of chocs and sweeties so temptingly displayed at hand height, perfect for quieting a squalling kiddie on the brink of throwing a tantrum.

Just take a look into the trolleys of your neighbours in the checkout queue. Like as not, you'll get an instant insight into couch potato land, a world where parent-child interaction amounts to little more than a constant demand and supply of fizzy pop and salty snacks.

There's big money to be made on these items: that big multi pack of crisps might look like good value, but if you were to crush it all down you'd end up with just a small heap of salty shavings. Sweets, crisps, cakes, fizzy drinks, high salt foods: these are all high margin items. Prices are constantly being shifted around, packaging re-designed, desires stimulated, all in the interest of boosting profits.

But if you're really paying attention, you can make the most of recent developments in labelling, checking out the dietary and nutritional information on the packs. There's still a long way to go in regulating supermarket practice, but we're not entirely at their mercy. What's going to make the difference is a bit of solid understanding of what different foods do to your body. That's where this book is going to be a big help.

Salt makes you fat and thirsty

Everyone needs salt, but it becomes a real problem when consumed in large quantities, way beyond what's good for us. For starters, it's going to make you thirsty. Walk into a pub and have a look at what snacks they are serving. Peanuts, crisps, pork scratchings . . . Why do they serve these salty foods? Of course, it's to make you buy more drinks. I'm sure you've already worked this out for yourself!

Just a small reduction in salt intake from 10 to 5 grams

per day would result in a reduction of essential daily fluid consumption by 350 ml. This is of particular significance when it comes to children, who are more likely to be quenching their salt-inspired thirst with their favourite fizzy drink. Cutting back on salt intake could make a major impact on childhood obesity.

Too much salt can cause the onset of chronic kidney disease, kidney stones, osteoarthritis, high blood pressure, stroke, heart disease and cancer. If you care about your health, give a thought to how much salt you are consuming. While you're at it, have a think about sodium. Salt (NaCl) is 40% sodium and 60% chloride. Examine the contents labels on prepackaged food and notice how many contain sodium. This is what you are looking to reduce. Keeping these sodium levels in check will make you less thirsty and ease your craving for those fizzy drinks and fruit juices. Foods to watch out for – foods best to avoid – include:

- Soups
- Cured meats
- Tomato sauce
- Pickles
- Processed cheese
- Condiments

Eating crap is addictive

If it was just a matter of keeping alert and well-informed it wouldn't be so difficult to stay on the strait and narrow, but the awkward fact is, that eating crap is addictive. It's one of the main reasons why we are getting fatter. The more crap we eat, resulting in an insulin spike, the more we crave, and the hungrier we feel. The body releases dopamine when we do something pleasurable, such as eating chocolate, snacking on crisps, eating junk food, smoking a fag, etc. It's a fix, and like all addictions, a tolerance builds up – you need more dopamine to get the same effect. It's a vicious cycle. No wonder our high streets are lined with fast food restaurants, because we're addicted to the junk they serve. Like all addictions, this is not going to be an easy habit to break, but if you do eat junk food regularly you definitely need to stop.

This book will have done its job if it helps you build the fierce resolve necessary to break those dangerous habits. It's really not good for your health or your waistline. It will be hard, but keep yourself well hydrated, stay focused and avoid these takeaway restaurants. You'll know it makes sense.

The economics of obesity & the cost to the NHS

It scares me how much obesity is costing the NHS. It's one of the main reasons why the overall cost of our health service has mushroomed in recent years. Estimates of the direct costs for treating excess weight, obesity and related morbidity have risen from £479.3 million in 1998 to £4.2 billion in 2007. Indirect costs (those costs arising from the impact of obesity on the wider economy, such as loss of productivity) over the same time period may well have risen from £2.6 billion to £15.8 billion. Modelled projections suggest that indirect costs could be as much as £27 billion by 2015.

In 2006/07, obesity and obesity-related illness was estimated to have cost £148 million for in-patient stays in

England. In Scotland, the total societal cost of obesity and overweight in 2007/08 was estimated to be between £600 million and £1.4 billion, of which the NHS may have contributed as much as £312 million.

Whilst these figures do suggest a significant overall increase in the costs of treating excess weight and obesity, it's worth bearing in mind that different studies have assessed and defined costs differently. This means it's hard to get a precise idea of the scale of the problem – but it is clear that it's a huge issue.

NHS tasks: estimated costs (£ millions)		
	1998	2002
Treating obesity	9.4	45.8-49.0
Treating consequences of obesity	469.9	945-1,075
Total direct costs	**479.3**	**990.8-1,124**
Lost earnings due to premature mortality	827.8	1,050-1,150
Lost earnings due to attributable sickness	1,321.7	1,300-1,450
Total indirect costs	**2,149.5**	**2,350-2,600**
Total economic cost of obesity	**2,628.9**	**3,340-3,724**

What does the future hold?

The statistical trends are alarming. Not only is the population growing at an unprecedented rate, but we are getting fatter and fatter.

From now (2016) to 2050 we will increase in number from 7 billion to over 9 billion.

Around 75% of the developed world will be overweight – that's going to be a huge problem. Literally.

Conditions associated with obesity

Obesity and being overweight are catalysts for other diseases and bodily disorders. The diagram below shows six of the most common associated conditions. The good news is that we can all do something about it.

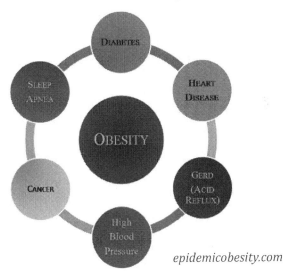

epidemicobesity.com

Our chances of developing these conditions diminish significantly just by improving our diet and exercising more. These are things we can directly influence, so why don't we do something about it? I think it's because we have grown lazy, comfortable with our bad habits. Now, habits form over many years, but they can be broken. New, good, habits can be established and encouraged. For example, why not get into the habit of exercising at least three times a week, following the principles and methods in this book? It's going to make a big difference in your life.

Diabetes (type 2)

The links between obesity and type 2 diabetes are firmly established: without the intervention of a healthy diet and exercise, obesity can lead to type 2 diabetes over a relatively short period of time. If you are overweight or obese, i.e. having a body mass index (BMI) of 30 or more, you face an 80-85% increased risk of developing this disease. Recent research suggests that obese people are up to 8 times more likely to develop type 2 diabetes than those with a BMI of less than 22. Think about it: your health is seriously at risk if you keep eating the way you do. We need to change our eating habits, before the NHS collapses under the burden of obesity.

Don't worry; there is some good news. Reducing your body weight, even by a small amount, can help improve your body's insulin sensitivity and lower your risk of developing cardiovascular and metabolic conditions such as type 2 diabetes, heart disease and some types of cancer. According to the NHS, just a 5% reduction in body weight followed up by regular moderate-intensity exercise could reduce your type 2 diabetes risk by more than 50%.

For example, let's say that you are 15 stone (210 lbs). If you followed the Nitro+ Diet and managed to lose just over 10 lbs you would have reduced your risk of developing type 2 diabetes by half. Yep, it's that easy. It's a proven fact: eating a healthy diet and exercising more can lower the risk of these conditions. Don't you think the time is right to change now? Not tomorrow, not next week or next month or after the holiday, DO IT NOW – your body, your family and the NHS will thank you for it.

Heart Disease / High Blood Pressure

Your heart is a muscle roughly the same size as a clenched fist. Every second of every day it keeps busily recycling your blood, constantly restoring your vigour. In the course of its journey round the arterial system, blood becomes depleted of oxygen; the heart receives this supply, pumping it into the lungs to become reoxygenated and cleansed of carbon dioxide. It's vitally important to keep your heart healthy.

Obesity can create big problems for your heart. Here's an analogy which should be familiar to anyone who's ever tended a garden in warm weather. Imagine a hosepipe that's pumping water onto your garden plants. What you would like is a continuous steady flow from the tap. If there's a kink in the hose, or you happen to step on it, water will no longer be discharging, but instead there'll be an increasing pressure on hosepipe and tap. If you allow this to continue, you may find that the pipe splits open, or springs free from the tap, resulting in a sudden catastrophic deluge.

The human body operates in a similar way, with the heart acting as the tap, and the veins and arteries as the hosepipe. What you want is a steady unrestricted flow, but diets high in fat can cause what is known as atherosclerosis, a potentially very serious condition in which the arteries become clogged up by fatty substances known as plaques or atheroma. The affected arteries become hard and narrow, restricting the flow of blood essential to keeping organs functioning healthily. This in turn will increase the blood pressure (just like in the constricted hosepipe) and cause more pressure on the heart. If a plaque ruptures, it can cause a blood clot, possibly triggering a heart attack, or, if blood supply to the brain becomes constricted, bringing on a stroke.

The risks faced by obese people of developing athero-sclerosis, coronary heart disease and congestive heart failure can be greatly reduced by restricting the amount of salt in your diet and by reducing excess weight.

Gerd (acid reflux / heartburn)

Oh my Gerd! Not many people know this, but it's the technical name for heartburn, or acid reflux, something you may be unlucky enough to have experienced.

Studies have shown that men and women who gain a few extra pounds can increase their risk of heartburn, whilst losing weight can reduce this likelihood. Although the causes of heartburn are not entirely understood, researchers surmise that extra fat around the belly increases the pressure on the stomach, loosening the restraining sphincter and forcing stomach acids up into the oesophagus (the gullet or foodpipe).

Being overweight can also slow down the body's ability to empty the stomach quickly. Researchers for the Nurse's Health Study, analyisng the health records of 10,000 women, found that a weight gain of 10 to 20 pounds was associated with a threefold increase in heartburn symptoms. When overweight tends toward obesity, the risk is inten-sified. Obese people are nearly three times more likely than normal weight people to have heartburn. The Nurse's Health Study concludes that losing weight can reduce a woman's risk of heartburn by as much as 40%.

Cancer

I hate cancer. It's had a big impact on my life. My dear old Mum was diagnosed with breast cancer in 2006, enduring treatment and a mastectomy. She was my rock, an amazing woman who would always say she felt fine, even in the darkest days of chemotherapy. When she lost her hair, she could still raise a laugh from me by answering the door in a pink punk rocker style wig! In 2012 my mum was signed off and it was confirmed she was free from cancer. She had finally got her life back, joined a rock choir and started exploring the world.

Then, just when we thought all was good, at the end of 2013 she started to complain of tiredness. The doctors reckoned that it was to do with coming off the cancer drugs that she'd been on for five years. After a couple of months things got worse: she developed a right-sided hand tremor and grew unsteady on her feet. We were told it could be low vitamin B_{12} – but she continued to deteriorate. Cancer was back, this time in a more aggressive form, in the brain. Sadly, she passed away at the beginning of July 2014 at the age of 68. I miss my mum everyday, and that's why I hate cancer.

What do we know about the connection between being overweight or obese and contracting cancer? It's about the harmful effects caused by excess body fat. Surplus fat produces hormones and proteins that can affect the way our cells work, as they are released into the bloodstream and circulated around the body. It can play havoc with the hormones – testosterone in men and oestrogen in women. Insulin levels in people who are overweight or obese also tend to increase; high insulin levels are a common feature of many cancers, although it's not clear if this plays a causative role.

More than one in twenty cases of cancer in the UK are thought to be linked to being overweight or obese. Types of cancer that are common in overweight or obese people include:

- Breast cancer (in women after the menopause)
- Bowel cancer
- Womb cancer
- Oesophageal cancer (food pipe)
- Gastric cardia cancer (a type of stomach cancer)
- Pancreatic cancer
- Kidney cancer
- Liver cancer
- (probably): gallbladder, ovarian and aggressive prostate cancers

This list of cancers includes two of the most common – breast and bowel – as well as three of the hardest to treat – pancreatic, oesophageal and gallbladder cancers.

Belly fat can be harmful

Not surprisingly, no one likes belly fat, but it's about so much more than whether you look good on the beach. Belly fat has all sorts of harmful consequences.

If you're excessively fat around the belly you are at more risk of developing kidney, oesophageal, pancreatic, breast and womb cancers. It's also worth bearing in mind that very young children who are considerably heavier than average may be storing up big problems: some studies have found that people who are overweight or obese as children have higher risks of developing some form of cancer later in life.

The trim figures and slim waists we might enjoy in our younger days gradually slip away as we meander into our middle age. Elasticated waistbands and shirts no longer neatly tucked in are a sure sign that body fat has started piling on. In men this tends to happen in the tummy area, whereas ladies are more likely to fill out around the hips, buttocks and the backs of the legs. As our mid sections grow, so do the health risks.

There are two different types of fat, subcutaneous and visceral. Subcutaneous fat is not so dangerous – this is the fat that lies beneath your skin, the stuff you can grasp between your fingers. Visceral fat, on the other hand, is more of a cause for concern, playing a role in a variety of health problems. It lies deeper within the belly cavity, nestling between our abdominal organs.

In women, visceral fat has been linked with breast and womb cancer and can lead to gallbladder complications resulting in surgery. It can cause metabolic disturbances and increase the risk of type 2 diabetes, cardiovascular disease and insulin resistance. Insulin resistance means that your body's muscle and liver cells don't react correctly to a normal burst of insulin, possibly bringing on type 2 diabetes.

There are many possible reasons why some people are prone to belly fat gain: it could be hormonal, or it may be that hereditary factors are responsible. Fat cells are biologically active, producing hormones and other substances that can affect your health by disrupting the normal hormonal balance and functioning.

Don't worry, all is not lost

The good news is that you can do something about it. You have the power to lower the risks, by changing your diet and by doing more exercise. A range of benefits will follow: lower blood pressure, reduced lower density cholesterol levels (bad cholesterol) and improved heart health.

The Nitro+ Diet and exercise program will burn body fat from head to toe, in particular that health-damaging visceral fat. By increasing your protein levels at the right times, consuming low glycaemic load carbohydrates and supplementation, as indicated in this book, you'll soon be shifting this belly fat at an impressive rate.

I recommend moderate exercise of at least 30-45 minutes per day. This could be going for a walk or a cycle ride, or taking your pooch around the park. When you combine this with the anabolic exercise workouts using the Bellmate Kinetic you'll notice how your body's fat burning engine ignites. It's amazing! I've seen so many people doing shedloads of sit-ups and crunches in the gym thinking it will make a difference to their belly fat, but I know it just isn't going to work. It will help strengthen and tighten the abdominal muscles but it won't do anything about deep visceral fat.

If you want to see your abs you'll need to burn the body fat that's covering them. A six pack is everyone's birthright – just allow the Nitro+ Diet to help you discover them.

Why don't traditional diets work?

Simple answer: they focus on weight loss, not fat loss.

They break down and strip off valuable muscle tissue, turning our bodies into inefficient catabolic machines. Remember, muscles are your fat-burning engines; fat is their fuel.

Weight loss is quick – but it won't be lasting! After a diet, weight is put back on just as quickly as you lost it and sometimes, just for good measure, additional weight is piled on so you end up even heavier than when you started.

This seems like a good point to introduce one of the special features of this book, the Nitro+ Principles. These are designed to act as essential guidelines for you, as you set about achieving rapid and lasting weight loss.

> *Nitro+ Principle # 1*
> **Forget all other diets that focus on weight loss**

Possible causes of obesity

Eating poor diets laden in fat and refined carbohydrates is bound to make you overweight or obese. However, some people may have a specific condition that can also cause obesity. I mention a few of the most common causes below. If you think you are showing symptoms of any of these, make an appointment to see your doctor and have it checked out.

Do you have you an underactive thyroid?

The thyroid is a gland located in the neck just below the Adam's apple. Its main job is to regulate the body's metabolic rate by producing hormones. Hypothyroidism is the condition in which not enough thyroid hormone is being produced. It occurs in approximately 1.5-2% of women and in 0.2% of men, becoming more common as we get older. Up to 10% of women over the age of 65 show some signs of this. The most common cause of adult hypothyroidism is Hashimoto's thyroiditis, which is caused by an autoimmunity disorder whereby the body produces antibodies that attack and gradually destroy the thyroid gland.

Women are eight times more likely than men to develop Hashimoto's thyroiditis, especially as they age. It can also run in families or be associated with genetic abnormalities such as Turner's syndrome, Klinefelter's syndrome, and Down's syndrome. It can be diagnosed with a blood test to check the levels of thyroid hormones in the blood. If this is detected it can be easily treated by taking daily hormone-replacement tablets called levothyroxine, which tops up the missing thyroxin hormone.

Are you insulin resistant?

Insulin resistance is when your muscles stop accepting signals from insulin, the hormone that enables you to metabolise sugar from carbohydrate. Now there's a problem: carbohydrates, instead of getting burnt off as energy, are stored away as fat, or packed off to the liver to be held there as glycogen. There's only so much glycogen that the liver can hold; when capacity is reached, fat synthesis is switched on – triglycerides are pumped out causing fat cells to expand, gradually filling up the liver. This condition is known as fatty liver.

Further likely consequences of insulin resistance include increased risk of type 2 diabetes, high blood pressure, increased triglycerides, reduced good cholesterol and increased body fat. This body fat is normally stored around the abdominal area. If you think you have any of these symptoms and are concerned you may be insulin resistant, be sure to have a word with your doctor. A simple blood test should be able to find out what's going on with your blood sugar levels.

Are you leptin resistant?

Blimey! We're really pushing the frontiers of knowledge! Leptin, isn't that the business where your fingers and toes start dropping off? Well, no, that's leprosy, which is something quite different. So what is it then? Should I be worried?

Lots of research has been done on leptin resistance and obesity, notably by Professor Robert H Lustig MD, professor of paediatrics at the University of California, San Francisco and a member of the Endocrine Society's Obesity Task Force. Leptin has been bandied around for decades as the fat or obese hormone, but actually it's more accurately described as our starvation hormone.

Leptin is a protein that's made in the fat cells, circulates in the bloodstream, and heads up to the hypothalamus, part of the brain which regulates the nervous system. "Leptin is the way your fat cells tell your brain that your energy thermostat is set right," says Lustig. It lets you know when you have enough stored energy in your fat cells to engage in normal, relatively inexpensive metabolic processes. If there's less food being eaten, either because you're on a diet, or if there's no food to be had, then less leptin gets produced. However, something worrying tends to happen when the individual is overweight or obese. Leptin resistance means we never get the message to stop eating, that sense that tells us, "I'm full, I've had enough". Instead, we continue shovelling it in and we carry on putting on weight.

Proper leptin function can be encouraged by cutting down on sugary foods, which will reduce insulin production and blood glucose fluctuations. Also, by moving away from a diet rich in refined carbohydrates: high levels of triglycerides, a.k.a. low density lipoprotein (LDL) choles-terols, can interfere with the body's messaging service, so we never get to hear that important message: "stop eating!"

MAXIM – the catalyst for fat loss

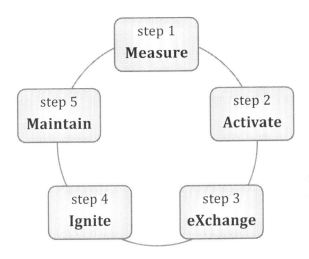

I'm a great believer in making things easy to follow, so I'm delighted to tell you that I've been able to condense all I have to say into a single watchword – MAXIM. It's a handy acronym for a code that you can live by, to make sure that you achieve the goal you've set for yourself: rapid and lasting weight loss, with you in the driving seat.

How to use this book

There are different ways you could set about this book. I've done my best to make it an interesting and entertaining read, so feel free to read it straight through, cover to cover. You're going to find out lots of useful stuff you probably never thought about before, and it'll be sure to set you thinking.

Alternatively, you could use it as a manual, dropping in on sections that sound promising. After all, no-one ever reads an automobile maintenance manual all the way through – or do they?

Personally, though, I would recommend reading the whole book, because it aims to present a systematic, reasoned argument which will build your understanding of the complex metabolic processes at work in the body, the end result of which is the body you wake up to every morning. There'll be a lot of science stuff, but you shouldn't need a Ph D to keep up. After you've finished, you'll be able to pull out the information you need to develop your very own personalised plan, before kicking off with the Nitro+ diet and exercise regime.

That's what it is, a plan, a system that will change your life for the better. For those of you who are intending to use this book as a manual there are some things that you need to have in place before you start the process. There are some supplements you may want to get hold of and you should also take a look at the exercises found in Step 4 – Ignite.

Here's a very short list of optional supplements you can order, ready for starting the Nitro+ Diet after Step 2 – Activate.

- Chromium   400 IU per day
- L - Carnitine   500 mg (tablets or powder)

Follow the MAXIM five step system and you will burn off body fat at an amazing rate – and it will stay off. This is not just a diet, it's a system. A system that takes you on a journey, and educates you along the way.

It's not designed for a quick fix. The MAXIM system will change the way you think about your body, inform you about the best things to eat and when, and teach you how to turn on your fat burning switch.

A short road map for your journey

The five step MAXIM system starts by measuring your body fat correctly and calculating your lean body mass (LBM), or in other words your fat free weight.

After you've taken this first step, it's time to activate and prepare your system with a detoxifying eating plan, which will last between two and four days depending on your lifestyle. This will allow the body to rid itself of its toxins and revitalise tired, overworked organs. It will establish the ideal environment to enable your energy system to switch from external to internal.

Now you'll be good and ready for the next stage – eXchange. This is where you start to create the perfect fat burning environment, confident that you're ingesting the ideal foods, at the ideal times, with the correct supplementation to kickstart your fat burning potential. You'll be at the controls: a diet of low glycaemic (GL) foods, in tandem with the healthy positive nitrogen balance produced by the change from catabolic to anabolic energy metabolism, will enable you to flick on the fat burning switch. That's it – those unwanted pounds of fat really are on the way out!

Throughout this book we'll be getting acquainted with some very important principles. These are going to be your friends and allies, helping you to get the most out of the Nitro+ Diet.

When we've succeeded in creating the perfect fat burning

environment we'll be ready for Step 4 – Ignite. This is where it starts to get really exciting: you'll have created the ideal environment for your body to make the switch from an external to an internal energy system.

This internal energy system is called gluconeogenesis. It's the process of using glucose from non-carbohydrate molecules, such as amino acids from protein or fatty acids from stored fats. Different supplements are introduced in order to crank up the metabolism, allowing the body to access more stored fat in order to transform it into energy.

You'll get to meet the innovative Bellmate Kinetic, your special partner for the exercise routines which form a key part of this programme. Resistance training two to three times per week will spark up the body's energy system, promoting good health and wellbeing while strengthening your bones and cardiovascular system. You'll find out about the best fat burning exercises and how to do them correctly to achieve optimal results.

Last and not least comes Step 5 – Maintain. This is what you'll be doing after you have reached your ideal weight and body composition. Carbohydrate intakes are increased, protein levels are dropped and maintenance supplements introduced to help inhibit the fat from coming back. Remember, with the Nitro+ Diet there'll be no backsliding.

Ok, are you ready? It starts here . . . the first step to a new you. Prepare to enjoy your new body – and Good Luck.

Case Study # 1 – Anna

"Sure, but will it work for me?" That's a fair question from anyone who's considering committing to some new "miracle diet". Well, I've been working with all sorts of people over many years, and I'd like to share some of the variety of transformations it's been my privilege to witness.

These Case Studies – six in all – will be appearing at the end of each chapter. They are all real people, although some of the names have been changed. The first concerns a 45 year old woman, "Anna".

Anna has had a history of trying out different diets. While these did initially help her to lose weight, after completing the diet all the weight would pile right back on.

From the initial assessment it was determined that Anna was severely dehydrated, with a low protein intake and a craving for sugars. Her muscles were in a negative nitrogen state.

The Nitro+ Diet was introduced, and she started going to the gym twice a week, doing mainly CV (cardiovascular) exercises on the bike, treadmill and cross trainer.

The chart on the next page shows how much difference just four weeks of following the Nitro+ Diet and exercise system made with this particular lady.

Before Nitro+ training	
Start weight:	155 lbs
Body fat %-age:	28%
Lean mass:	112 lbs
Fat mass:	43 lbs
Category:	Overweight
After four weeks	
Weight:	145 lbs
Body fat %-age:	20%
Lean mass:	116 lbs
Fat mass:	29 lbs
Category:	Normal

These results bear impressive testimony to the Nitro+ system. In just four weeks, not only had 10 lbs in overall weight fallen away, but also the fat to muscle ratio had significantly improved: an estimated 14 pounds fat loss combined with a 4 pound increase in muscle mass.

Energy levels were higher throughout the diet period, allowing resistance training to be introduced 3 times per week, with intervals added to her CV routine.

Anna wanted a diet that worked – to lose weight for good. Happily, the fat she lost has stayed lost.

So, now we're going to explore in detail how the process works, in five easy steps.

Step 1-Measure

Move over BMI: Lean Body Mass is king!

What makes Lean Body Mass (LBM) so important? Traditionally, Body Mass Index (BMI) has been used as the standard benchmark for planning exercise regimes, but it really doesn't cut the mustard. BMI is not an accurate measurement for fat and doesn't help us understand the causes of poor health.

A person's BMI is a number obtained by dividing their weight in kilograms by their height in metres, then squaring the result. It goes back a long way, 185 years in fact, having been created by the Belgian mathematician, astronomer and sociologist Lambert Adolphe Jacques Quetlet (1796-1874), but it seems like time to let it go. The fact is, BMI is actually not a good way to measure health.

It seems mad to me that we are still using this out of date metric. BMI doesn't take into account fat, muscle tissue or your body type, nor does it indicate where fat is distributed on the body. For instance, when belly fat increases so does the risk of diabetes, heart disease and death, whereas peripheral or subcutaneous fat (fat beneath the skin elsewhere in the body) may be harmless. It also doesn't allow for differences in race, gender, age and genetics. It leaves taller people thinking they are fatter than they actually are and shorter people thinking they are thinner – rather like a distorting mirror at the fairground. There are other ways to measure body fat out there that are much more useful and reliable.

Some techniques can require sophisticated gadgetry, such as MRI, CT and DEXA scans; understandably, these can work out quite expensive. At the other end of the scale, an easy way to detect possible type 2 diabetes and cardiovascular diseases is by calculating your waist to height ratio. Keeping your waist circumference to less than half your height is a great way to increase your life expectancy.

My own favourite method involves using fat callipers to measure fat at various (between four and seven) points on the body: we'll be looking at this in detail in a short while. It's a method that calculates the visceral fat – the fat that's sandwiched in between your internal organs, which can raise your risk of type 2 diabetes and cardio-vascular disease. Visceral fat develops deep among muscles and around organs like the liver; by releasing certain hormones and other agents, it disrupts the body's ability to balance its energy needs. The amount of fat that gathers around your waist is a particularly helpful indicator of general health, since tummy fat affects the heart, liver and kidneys more than, for example, fat distributed around your hips and bottom.

Measuring your Lean Body Mass

Lean Body Mass (LBM) is a much more accurate measurement when it comes to knowing how much fat you are carrying. LBM is an index of body composition, calculated by subtracting body fat weight from total body weight: total body weight is lean plus fat.

We can formulate this using the following equation:

> **Lean Body Mass = Body Weight − Body Fat**
> *Or:* **LBM = BW − BF**

The percentage of total body mass that is lean is usually not quoted – it would typically be between 60 and 90%. Instead, the body fat percentage – the total mass of fat divided by total body mass – is the figure normally cited; generally this lies between 10 and 40%. Lean body mass (LBM) has particular advantages over total body weight when it comes to assessing metabolic disorders and determining appropriate medication levels, since overall body fat is less relevant for metabolic processes.

How to measure body fat percentage (BFP)

Let's look at how you find out your body fat percentage. It's an important thing to know: from this information you can find out your own lean body mass, allowing you to calculate how much protein, carbohydrates and fats you need on a daily basis. You can also monitor your progress with the Nitro+ Diet to see how much fat has been lost.

If you go to our website, *www.bellmatesystems.com,* you can use our FREE Nitro+ Diet calculator. Just click on the drop down and select your preferred method of calculation, then leave the rest to us. ☺

There are many methods out there to measure body fat. Some are better than others. These are my top three:

1.   Fat Callipers

This is my favourite, and is the most accurate, way to measure body fat. Measurements are taken at up to seven points on the body, using a gadget that looks like something from a 1950s sci-fi movie.

And where can I get these instruments? Just type "body fat callipers" into your search engine – they'll only cost you a couple of quid – it's a great investment!

The best time to measure fat is before breakfast, first thing in the morning. The following descriptions relate to measurements taken on the right hand side of the body, as is conventional.

Pectoral (chest):

The pinch is taken at approximately one third of the distance from the armpit to the nipple, at a diagonal to the nipple-armpit line.

Abdomen (belly):

A vertical or horizontal fold is taken two centimetres to the right of the bellybutton (umbilicus). Most people find that the fat folds easier with a vertical pinch, but feel free to use the most comfortable direction for you.

Quadriceps (thigh):

The skin fold here should be taken in the front, halfway between the upper part of the knee (the proximal patella, where it corners when the leg is bent) and the fold above the thigh when the leg is raised (the inguinal fold). The vertical fold will need to be pinched a little harder, since fat and skin tissue in this area tends to be somewhat firmer, and in consequence the thigh skin fold may over-estimate fat content.

Triceps (upper arm, back):

Pinch a vertical skin fold halfway down the upper arm. If you want to be more precise, use a tape between the bony top of the shoulder or acromial (do not confuse it with the bony upper part of the shoulder blade!) and the most prominent tip of the elbow (radial). Mark a dot or a horizontal line at half the measured distance; this is where the vertical fat fold should be pinched.

Subscapular (shoulder blade, lower tip):

Raise the outline of the shoulder blade (scapula) by carefully moving the arm behind the back, and note the position of the bottom corner of the shoulder blade. Replace the arm to resting position, then pinch the skin approximately two centimetres below this bottom corner, at an angle of 45°, more or less parallel to the inside angle of the shoulder blade.

Suprailiac or iliac crest (hip, front):

The iliac crest is the top ridge of your hip bone. This skin fold is right below the front or anterior part of the armpit (axilla). From here follow a vertical line until you meet the hipbone. The skin fold is an angled one (roughly 45°, heading away from the groin), about two centimetres above the iliac crest. The fold spot should be between the top of the hipbone on the side and the bony part on the lower right of the belly (which is still part of the same hipbone), following the natural fold of the skin.

Midaxillary (armpit at fifth rib):

This fold is taken on the side of the torso, either horizontally or vertically (though most commonly vertically), at the fifth rib. Fifth rib position can be determined by locating the lower tip of the breast bone (xiphoid process) and following a horizontal line to the side of the torso until you're right below the armpit (axilla). The arm should be raised at approximately chest height.

2. Fat Percentage Scales

These are growing in popularity, having become much more affordable than they used to be. The scales are very simple to use and give you a fairly accurate measurement, give or take 1-2% – not quite as accurate as the skin fold method.

I can recommend the Omron HBF 510 Body Composition Monitor with Scale, which is one of the most accurate, retailing at around £50-£60. It will calculate your body fat percentage, lean body fat mass and weight either in pounds (lbs) or kilograms (kgs).

3. Lean Body Mass calculation

Ok, this is slightly different: with this measurement you go straight to your lean body mass, which is after all what we're aiming for. It's usually estimated using one of three possible mathematical formulas. The following formula is the least precise, but it will give you a rough idea if you don't have a set of callipers or fat percentage scales to hand.

You will need to know your weight in kilograms and your height in centimetres. Remember, one kilogram is equivalent to 2.2 pounds.

LBM calculation: for men
LBM = (0.32810 x W) + (0.33929 x H) − 29.5336
LBM calculation: for women
LBM = (0.29569 x W) + (0.41813 x H) − 43.2933

W: body weight in kilograms   H: body height in centimetres

When you know your lean body mass the rest is a doddle. If you want to know your lean body mass in pounds, just remember to multiply by 2.2.

Knowing your LBM allows you to calculate your optimal daily consumption of protein, using the following equations.

Calculating optimal daily protein intake
For women: LBM x 0.8 = grams of protein per day   **For men:**   LBM = grams of protein per day

Basic principle

Men: Consume 1 gram of protein for every pound of LEAN body weight

Women: Consume 0.8 grams of protein for every pound of LEAN body weight.

Men get a particularly easy ride here! Women will need to multiply their LBM by 0.8 (i.e. calculate 80%).

Calorific content of different food types

Protein	4 calories per gram
Carbohydrates	4 calories per gram
Fats	9 calories per gram

Calories are a measure of the potential energy in food. Different categories of food vary in their calorific content, as you can see in the table above. Protein and carbohydrates both contribute four calories per gram, whilst the calorific content of fat is more than double this, at nine calories per gram.

Knowing your optimum protein levels will allow you to work out how to calculate your daily requirements for carbohydrates and fats.

How to work out your daily intake of proteins, carbohydrates and fats for purposes of fat loss

The effectiveness of the Nitro+ Diet in promoting fat loss depends on its high levels both of protein and low glycaemic carbohydrates.

The Nitro+ Diet formula is:

Proteins	30%
Carbohydrates (intact slow digesting)	50%
Fats (unsaturated)	20%

At this point, you should know your bodyweight, height, body-fat and your unique Lean Body Mass number (LBM). Once you have this number you will be able to work out how much protein you need on a daily basis.

It's going to help if you have a calculator handy. To work out the carbohydrates and fats, use the following calculations.

Nitro+ Diet ideal nutrition

Protein (grams) – men:	LBM number
Protein (grams) – women:	Multiply LBM x 0.8
Carbohydrates (grams):	Multiply LBM x 1.67
Fats (grams):	Multiply LBM x 0.3

I'm going to give you some examples to help get you into the swing of things. First of all, there's a couple involving women. A word of warning here: you might notice that body weights are given in pounds, while protein intake is measured in grams. Well, that's how they work it stateside, and it's generally not a problem. But, if I were designing a rocket ship, I'd definitely want to be paying close attention.

Example one: female

A woman weighs 200 lbs, with a body fat of 38% (thus, a lean mass percentage of 62%). First we'll calculate her lean body mass, in terms of pounds, then we'll work out the appropriate protein intake:

200 (weight in lbs) **x 0.62** (lean mass percentage)

= 124 lbs (LBM)

x 0.8 (adjustment for women)

= 99.2 (i.e. 99 grams of protein)

Now we'll be able to calculate appropriate daily levels of protein, carbohydrates and fats:

Total Protein:		=	99 grams
Total Carbs:	99 x 1.67	=	165 grams
Total Fats:	99 x 0.3	=	29.7 grams
Calculating appropriate daily calorie intake			
Proteins:	99 x 4	=	396 calories
Carbohydrates:	165 x 4	=	660 calories
Fats:	29.7 x 9	=	267 calories
Total daily calories		**=**	**1,323 calories**

Example two: female

A woman weighs 180 lbs and a has a body fat of 40%. To calculate her lean body mass, we'll follow the same process as above:

180 (weight in lbs) **x 0.60** (lean mass percentage)

= 108 lbs (LBM)

x 0.8 (adjustment for women)

= 86.4 (i.e. 86.4 grams of protein)

Calculating appropriate daily levels of protein, carbohydrates and fats:

Total Protein:		=	86.4 grams
Total Carbs:	86.4 x 1.67	=	144 grams
Total Fats:	86.4 x 0.3	=	26 grams

Calculating appropriate daily calorie intake

Proteins:	86.4 x 4	=	345.6 calories
Carbohydrates:	144 x 4	=	576 calories
Fats:	26 x 9	=	234 calories
Total daily calories		**=**	**1,155.6 calories**

In case all this maths has left you feeling a bit lost in a wilderness of numbers, you might like to use our FREE NITRO+ CALCULATOR at *www.bellmatesystems.com*.

Alternatively, you could use the following chart as a guide. Weights are presented in increments of 10 lbs, going from 120 to 250 lbs, with a range of body fat percentages (from 20-40%) given for each weight.

It's handy, but I do recommend that you work out your own unique LBM, in order to get the most out of the Nitro+ Diet method.

Nutritional guidelines for women

Weight (lbs)	Body fat %	Body fat (lbs)	LBM (lbs)	Protein (g)	Carbs (g)	Fats (g)	Calories
120	40	48	72	58	97	17	773
120	35	42	78	62	104	18	826
120	30	36	84	67	112	20	896
120	25	30	90	72	120	21	957
120	20	24	96	77	129	23	1031
130	40	52	78	62	104	18	826
130	35	46	84	68	114	20	908
130	30	39	91	73	122	21	969
130	25	33	97	78	130	23	1039
130	20	26	104	83	139	24	1104
140	40	56	84	67	112	20	896
140	35	49	91	73	122	21	969
140	30	42	98	78	130	23	1039
140	25	35	105	84	140	25	1121
140	20	28	112	90	150	26	1194
150	40	60	90	72	120	21	957
150	35	53	98	78.4	130	23	1040.6
150	30	45	105	84	140	25	1121
150	25	37.5	113	90.4	150	26	1195.6
150	20	30	120	96	160	28	1276
160	40	64	96	77	129	23	1031
160	35	56	104	83	139	24	1104
160	30	48	112	90	150	26	1194
160	25	40	120	96	160	28	1276
160	20	32	128	102	171	30	1362
170	40	68	102	82	137	24	1092
170	35	60	111	88	148	26	1178
170	30	51	119	95	159	28	1268

Weight (lbs)	Body fat %	Body fat (lbs)	LBM (lbs)	Protein (g)	Carbs (g)	Fats (g)	Calories
170	25	43	128	102	170	30	1358
170	20	34	136	109	182	32	1452
180	40	72	108	86	144	25	1145
180	35	63	117	94	157	28	1256
180	30	54	126	101	169	30	1350
180	25	45	135	108	180	32	1440
180	20	36	144	115	192	34	1534
190	40	76	114	91	152	27	1215
190	35	67	123	99	165	29	1317
190	30	57	133	106	177	31	1411
190	25	48	142	114	190	33	1511
190	20	38	152	122	204	36	1628
200	40	80	120	96	160	28	1276
200	35	70	130	104	174	31	1391
200	30	60	140	112	187	33	1493
200	25	50	150	120	200	35	1595
200	20	40	160	128	214	38	1710
210	40	84	126	100	168	30	1342
210	35	74	136	109	182	32	1452
210	30	63	147	118	197	35	1575
210	25	53	157	126	210	37	1677
210	20	42	168	134	224	39	1783
220	40	88	132	106	177	31	1411
220	35	77	143	114	190	33	1513
220	30	66	154	123	205	36	1636
220	25	55	165	132	220	39	1759
220	20	44	176	141	235	41	1873
230	40	92	138	110	184	32	1464
230	35	81	149	119	199	35	1587
230	30	69	161	129	215	38	1718

Weight (lbs)	Body fat %	Body fat (lbs)	LBM (lbs)	Protein (g)	Carbs (g)	Fats (g)	Calories
230	25	58	172	138	230	40	1832
230	20	46	184	147	245	43	1955
240	40	96	144	115	192	34	1534
240	35	84	156	125	209	37	1669
240	30	72	168	134	224	39	1782
240	25	60	180	144	240	42	1916
240	20	48	192	154	257	45	2050
250	40	100	150	120	200	35	1595
250	35	88	162	130	217	38	1730
250	30	75	175	140	234	42	1874
250	25	63	187	150	251	44	2000
250	20	50	200	160	267	47	2131

Example three: male

A man weighs 260 lbs and has a body fat of 40%. We can calculate his lean body mass, then determine the appropriate nutritional levels:

260 (weight in lbs) **x 0.60** (lean mass percentage) **= 156 lbs** (LBM)

Total Protein:		=	156 grams
Total Carbs:	156 x 1.67	=	260.5 grams
Total Fats:	156 x 0.3	=	46.8 grams

Calculating appropriate daily calorie intake

Proteins:	156 x 4	=	624 calories
Carbohydrates:	260.5 x 4	=	1,042 calories
Fats:	46.8 x 9	=	421 calories
Total daily calories		**=**	**2,087 calories**

Example four: male

A man weighs 180 lbs and has a 25% level of body fat. To discover his lean body mass:

180 (weight in lbs) **x 0.75** (lean mass percentage)
= 135 lbs (LBM)

We can now calculate appropriate daily levels of protein, carbohydrates and fats:

Total Protein:		=	135 grams
Total Carbs:	135 x 1.67	=	225.5 grams
Total Fats:	135 x 0.3	=	40.5 grams

Calculating appropriate daily calorie intake

Proteins:	135 x 4	=	540 calories
Carbohydrates:	225.5 x 4	=	902 calories
Fats:	40.5 x 9	=	364.5 calories
Total daily calories		**=**	**1,806.5 calories**

Now here's another handy chart, this time for men, so you can check if you're on the right track. Remember, you need to measure your body fat first in order to find out your lean body mass (LBM). When you know your LBM you can calculate your nutritional daily intake.

> **Lean body percentage**
>
> **= 100 − body fat percentage**

Nutritional guidelines for men

Weight (lbs)	Body fat %	Body fat (lbs)	LBM (lbs)	Protein (g)	Carbs (g)	Fats (g)	Calories
150	40	60	90	90	150	26	1194
150	35	52	98	98	163	29	1305
150	30	45	105	105	175	31	1399
150	25	37	113	113	189	33	1505
150	20	30	120	120	200	35	1595
160	40	64	96	96	160	28	1276
160	35	56	104	104	174	31	1391
160	30	48	112	112	187	33	1493
160	25	40	120	120	200	35	1595
160	20	32	128	128	214	38	1710
170	40	68	102	102	170	30	1358
170	35	60	110	110	184	32	1464
170	30	51	119	119	199	35	1587
170	25	43	127	127	212	37	1689
170	20	34	136	136	227	40	1812
180	40	72	108	108	180	32	1440
180	35	63	117	117	195	34	1554
180	30	54	126	126	210	37	1677

Weight (lbs)	Body fat %	Body fat (lbs)	LBM (lbs)	Protein (g)	Carbs (g)	Fats (g)	Calories
180	25	45	135	135	225	40	1800
180	20	36	144	144	240	42	1914
190	40	76	114	114	190	33	1513
190	35	67	123	123	205	36	1636
190	30	57	133	133	222	39	1771
190	25	48	142	142	237	42	1894
190	20	38	152	152	254	45	2029
200	40	80	120	120	200	35	1595
200	35	70	130	130	217	38	1730
200	30	60	140	140	234	41	1865
200	25	50	150	150	251	44	2000
200	20	40	160	160	267	47	2131
210	40	84	126	126	210	37	1677
210	35	74	137	137	229	41	1833
210	30	63	147	147	245	43	1955
210	25	53	157	157	262	47	2099
210	20	42	168	168	281	49	2237
220	40	88	132	132	220	39	1759
220	35	77	143	143	239	42	1906
220	30	66	154	154	257	45	2049
220	25	55	165	165	276	48	2196
220	20	44	176	176	294	52	2348
230	40	92	138	138	230	40	1832
230	35	81	149	149	249	44	1988
230	30	69	161	161	267	47	2135
230	25	58	172	172	287	50	2286
230	20	46	184	184	307	54	2450
240	40	96	144	144	240	42	1914
240	35	84	156	156	261	46	2082
240	30	72	168	168	281	49	2237

Weight (lbs)	Body fat %	Body fat (lbs)	LBM (lbs)	Protein (g)	Carbs (g)	Fats (g)	Calories
240	25	60	180	180	301	53	2401
240	20	48	192	192	321	56	2556
250	40	100	150	150	251	44	2000
250	35	88	162	162	271	48	2164
250	30	75	175	175	292	51	2327
250	25	63	187	187	312	55	2491
250	20	50	200	200	334	59	2667
260	40	104	156	156	261	46	2082
260	35	91	169	169	282	50	2254
260	30	78	182	182	304	53	2421
260	25	65	195	195	326	57	2597
260	20	52	208	208	347	61	2769
270	40	108	162	162	271	48	2164
270	35	95	175	175	292	51	2327
270	30	81	189	189	316	55	2515
270	25	68	202	202	337	59	2687
270	20	54	216	216	361	63	2875
280	40	112	168	168	281	49	2237
280	35	98	182	182	304	53	2421
280	30	84	196	196	327	57	2605
280	25	70	210	210	351	62	2802
280	20	56	224	224	374	66	2986

What's so special about the Nitro+ Diet?

Yes, it is true that high protein, high fat, low carbohydrate diets do burn body fat. Many diets working on these principles have been best sellers, but – watch out! – they can lead to big problems. Large quantities of the wrong proteins and saturated fat (high fat meats, bacon etc) could have the following unwished-for results:

- High cholesterol: a consequence of large amounts of fatty meats, whole dairy and other high fat foods.
- Kidney problems: excessive amounts of protein can put added strain on the kidneys, leading to deteriorating kidney function and the development of kidney stones.
- Osteoporosis: eating very high levels of protein may result in urinating more calcium than normal, which could make osteoporosis worse.

These problems, all associated with protein levels in excess of 35% total calorie intake, may also bring on the dangerous conditions of hyperaminoacidemia, hyperammonemia, and hyperinsulinemia, not to mention nausea and diarrhoea.

Low carbohydrate diets may also result in ketosis – a metabolic state dependent on ketone bodies (rather than blood glucose) for energy, which can, if the ketone levels become sufficiently high, trigger ketoacidosis.

Not to worry if the medical terminology doesn't make much sense to you; the main message I'd like you to take on board is this:

> **Don't eat too much protein
> – it's really not good for you.**

For men, one gram of protein per pound of lean body mass is the right level of protein for switching the body's fat burning engine on and the catabolic switch off. For women, the equivant amount is 0.8 grams. Once you're equipped with this information, you become the Controller.

Safe and sure

The Nitro+ Diet has been designed to be worry-free, advocating a daily calorie intake obtained from no more than 30% protein and 50% low GL carbohydrates. It's a very safe diet to follow, without the disturbing side effects associated with other diets. You'll be astonished how the fat simply melts away, even while you're eating plenty of food throughout the day. I've witnessed some amazing transformations!

If you stick to the diet, it will work. If you're not experiencing the promised effects, then you need to work just a bit harder, to be sure of creating the right exercise and metabolic environments. The Nitro+ Diet guarantees a fantastic, safe, fat burning process as well as encouraging healthy gluconeogenesis, the process of making glucose from non-carbohydrate foods such as protein and fats. Although there will be times in this diet when your body switches into mild ketosis (for example, after sleeping and between meals) this will not be constant. Instead, the Nitro+ Diet system works by maintaining a positive nitrogen balance. Your fat burning switch is activated, turning your muscles into fat burning furnaces.

Case Study # 2 – Beth

"Beth" was a 23 year old woman, particularly concerned about her weight around the hips, thighs and gluteal area.

The Nitro+ Diet was introduced with a 5 day detox plan to kick it off. She started training with light weights with a rep range of 15 x 3 sets, 3 times per week.

Before Nitro+ training	
Start weight:	216 lbs
Body fat %-age:	33%
Lean mass:	145 lbs
Fat mass:	71 lbs
Category:	Obese
After four weeks	
Weight:	205 lbs
Body fat %-age:	28%
Lean mass:	148 lbs
Fat mass:	57 lbs
Category:	Above average

The total weight lost was 11 pounds, but what is really impressive here is the changing ratio of fat to lean mass. Body fat decreased by an amazing 5% – 14 lbs of fat burned off! – while muscle mass increased by 3 lbs.

Not only had weight training increased muscle mass, but her muscles had switched into a positive nitrogen balance.

A fantastic result for Beth – and for the Nitro+ Diet.

Step 2-Activate

Preparing the system

Are you tired all the time?

To get the best from the Nitro+ Diet the body needs to be prepared. It's like when you're setting about doing some home improvement – repainting the walls in your living room, say. Before you get busy slapping on the chosen topcoat, you (or your decorator) need to take some time on the prep: first of all protecting the rest of the stuff in the room from inadvertent paint splashes, then cleaning the surfaces to be painted, filling in any holes, deciding whether you need an undercoat . . . By the time you eventually prise open your chosen shade of Passion Red and let that colour spread across the walls, you can be confident you're going to end up with the best, most durable result.

Just so with the body: we need to prime, prepare and activate the system before attempting a major overhaul of its operating conditions.

Take care of your small intestine

After your food passes through the stomach, digestion is completed in the small intestine. This can get bunged up, particularly as a consequence of eating meat, which tends to take longer to digest than other foods. Detoxing will help flush the intestines through.

Your small intestine is approximately five meters in length and is the longest section of your digestive tract – longer than your large intestine, although with a smaller diameter. In the course of digestion, food is propelled through the small intestine by the process of peristalsis, a pulsing muscular movement alternating contraction and relaxation. We've all experienced times when this process can feel difficult or uncomfortable. The good news is that movement and exercise can greatly assist peristaltic action and generally aid digestion.

The small intestine manages to absorb most of our nutrients by means of a very fine mesh on its inside wall, composed of membranous protrusions known as microvilli. Each individual microvillus contains a tiny blood capillary, and is packed with enzymes enabling the breakdown of complex nutrients into more readily absorbed compounds. These are then passed into the bloodstream, the body's built-in nutrient distribution system, to be circulated to the vital organs, muscles, etc – wherever they're needed. The mass of stuff left over after this extraction process then gets propelled through your large intestine and eventually out into the dunny.

It's a very good idea not to make things difficult for the small intestine. For example, eating a diet high in refined carbohydrates and saturated fat – the mainstay of fast food – can leave you really exhausted, as well as prone to type 2 diabetes and hypoglycaemia. The adrenal / pancreas / thyroid axis is constantly under tremendous stress, forced to work overtime. The result is continual rides on the blood glucose and insulin rollercoaster, which really takes its toll on the body.

I'm going to dip into a little bit of science to help you to understand how poor diets can affect these glands and lead to possible symptoms of dysfunction. I've tried to make it easy to follow, so do stick with it – it'll be worth the effort.

Adrenal glands

These are around the size of a walnut and are located at the top of your kidneys. Adrenal gland dysfunction is nowadays very common, and is a major factor in causing a thyroid hormone imbalance.

The adrenal glands produce many hormones, including DHEA (from cholesterol) and cortisol. DHEA is a sex hormone, a great immune system enhancer and is anabolic (remember, anabolic is about building things up, the opposite of catabolic). Cortisol slows down digestion, can suppress immune function and will raise blood sugar levels if we are under stress. It's sometimes known as our fight or flight hormone.

Common symptoms of adrenal gland dysfunctions include:

- Blurred vision
- Bloatedness
- Craving for caffeine or cigarettes

- Dizziness
- Fatigue
- Allergies
- Weakened immune system
- Ulcers
- Haemorrhoids
- Asthma
- Salt or sugar cravings
- Headaches
- Varicose veins
- Insomnia

Pancreas

The pancreas is around six inches long and plays a very important role in the digestive system. It's located within the upper abdomen and is surrounded by the stomach, small intestine, liver and spleen. The pancreas is pear shaped and produces digestive juices and enzymes to assist in the digestion of fats and proteins. More importantly, it also produces the hormone insulin (together with other hormones) that controls blood sugar levels. Insulin is released when blood sugar is increased. It's a decision maker, causing muscles and other tissues to take up glucose from the blood.

Common symptoms of a pancreatic disorder are:

- Diarrhoea
- Pain in the stomach (upper abdomen)
- Back pain
- Jaundice (yellowing of skin and eyes)
- Nausea
- Bloating
- Vomiting

Pancreatic exhaustion and failure

Eating an unhealthy diet loaded with sugars and fats can cause pancreatic dysfunction. Eating too much sugar, whether in candies, cookies, cakes, or even bread and pasta, can result in sugar overload. As the body sets about breaking down these sugars in the process of digestion, the resulting blood sugar imbalances can lead to diseases such as diabetes. The rapid alternation between high and low blood sugar levels associated with diabetes leads to the deterioration of the pancreas and eventually pancreatic exhaustion. All this can be prevented by following a proper diet.

Because the main job of the pancreas is to regulate blood sugar, pancreatic exhaustion is common amongst diabetics. After so much hard work struggling to bring down an overload of sugar, it can stop producing insulin hormones altogether, making it impossible for the body to break down sugar at all. This is why diabetics need to check their insulin levels on a regular basis, topping up their insulin with injections whenever necessary.

Thyroid

The thyroid gland is a butterfly shaped endocrine gland located at the front of your neck, just below your Adam's apple. It's made up of two lobes – the right lobe and the left lobe, each about the size of a plum cut in half – joined by a small bridge of thyroid tissue called the isthmus. The two lobes lie on either side of your windpipe.

Two important hormones – thyroxin (T4) and triiodothyronine (T3) – are secreted by the thyroid gland into the bloodstream. We need these hormones for all the cells in the body to function normally. Thyroid disorders are very common; women are particularly susceptible, although anyone – men, teenagers, children and babies too – can be affected. About one in twenty people (5%) have some kind of thyroid disorder, either temporary or permanent.

The thyroid also produces thyroid hormone (TH), which regulates, among other things, your body's temperature, metabolism, and heartbeat. Problems can arise from both hyperactivity – producing too much TH – and sluggishness – the production of too little TH, a condition known as hypothyroidism.

Foods that can cause hypothyroidism

An underactive thyroid, or hypothyroidism, can be caused by some foods, especially if you have an iodine deficiency. These foods are known as goitrogens because they can trigger the enlargement of the thyroid (a goitre) as well as hypothyroidism. They block the conversion of T4 hormone to T3, the active form of thyroid hormone. Among the more common foods that cause this condition are:

- Almond seeds
- Brussels sprouts
- Cabbage
- Cauliflower
- Corn (maize)
- Kale
- Turnips

Liver

It is estimated that 75% of obese people are likely to have a fatty liver. How does fat get into the liver? Well, metabolising fat is the liver's job, but if you eat too much saturated fat it stays stored in the liver cells, causing them to swell up.

Carrying excess abdominal fat is associated with fatty liver disease, as well as other conditions such as diabetes and heart trouble. For men, these risks increase if your waistline measures more than 102cm (40"); for women, the corresponding figure is 88cm (35") or more. You need to keep an eye on this: the more holes you have to add on your belt, the higher the risk!

Worryingly, there is no medication proven to be effective in treating fatty liver disease when this is related to obesity, diabetes or dyslipidaemia. However, it is possible for obese patients suffering from a fatty liver to reduce liver inflammation by bringing down their bodyweight by 10-20% through proper nutrition and exercise. So there is something you can do about it.

It's time to stop moaning about how you look and making up excuses as to why you can't get to the gym or eat healthily; if you want to make the most of your short span of life on this planet, it's worth giving some careful attention to the sort of food that you're eating.

Just how healthy are you?

We live in a very hectic world, constantly on the move. We're surrounded by 'smart' electronics, bombarding us with invisible waves and signals from microwaves, mobile phones, wifi etc. This is actually not good for you; it may be compromising your immune system.

The immune system is something that most of us take for granted. It allows us to operate freely in the world, relatively untroubled by the swirling soup of microbiological agents that swarm around in our atmosphere and environment. It's always switched on, ready for action.

The interlinked networks of cells, tissues and organs that comprise our bodies all have a share in the immune system, working together synergistically to maintain and protect the whole, but special honour must be paid to the white blood cells (leukocytes) which cruise the blood-stream, seeking out and destroying disease-causing organisms or substances.

Coming up on the next page are a few questions for you to consider. Be honest with your answers and you'll be able to see how your immune system shapes up.

Feel free to use a pen or pencil to indicate whether your answer is a Yes or a No. You'll be scoring 1 for a Yes answer, 0 for a No.

20 questions about your immune system

Score

1 Is your normal diet high in processed and / or sugary foods? . . . .

2 Do you eat fast food more than twice per week? . . . .

3 Do you have amalgam dental fillings? . . . .

4 Do you eat bread? . . . .

5 Do you always feel tired or under the weather? . . . .

6 Do you suffer from frequent colds or flu? . . . .

7 Do you suffer from stomach problems / wind / indigestion? . . . .

8 Do you exercise less than twice per week? . . . .

9 Do you sleep for less than eight hours a night? . . . .

10 Do you drink more than 2 diet drinks per week? . . . .

11 Do you eat red meat more than twice per week? . . . .

12 Do you feel constantly stressed and find it hard to concentrate? . . . .

13 Do you skip breakfast? . . . .

14 Do you regularly drink fruit juice or fizzy pop? . . . .

15 Do you smoke? . . . .

16 Do you drink alcohol more than 2 days per week? . . . .

17 Do you have teeth marks around your tongue? . . . .

18 Do you use a computer / games console / smart-phone daily? . . . .

19 Do you use a microwave daily? . . . .

20 Do you drink tea or coffee daily? . . . .

How did you score? **Your total** . . . .

15-20	health / immunity is poor	4 days detox
10-15	health / immunity is average	3 days detox
Below 10	health / immunity is good	2 days detox

So, how did you manage? Do you feel the need to improve your health and immunity?

It's your great good fortune that you can do something about it. Just follow the Nitro+ Diet activation programme, and you'll be able to work with your body as it restores its natural defences.

First of all I recommend a few days detox, depending on your result. For those scoring highest, indicating poor health and immunity, four days detox are advisable. Average scores merit three days, lowest scores just two.

The Nitro+ Diet Activation Programme

Before any change of nutritional plan I always recommend a detox to allow the body to remove any toxins, flush through the digestive system to improve absorption in the small intestines and generally nourish the internal organs. This process will cleanse the body and create a sound foundation for good health, which you can then build upon.

The Nitro+ Diet Activation Programme consists of fresh fruit and vegetables, with NO stimulants. These foods are naturally alkalising, and are thus helpful to excessively acid constitutions by neutralising accumulated stomach acid. The reduced calorie intake will also help burn up excess body fat.

As well as needing to eject unwanted chemicals absorbed from the atmosphere or in food and drink, the body also, in the course of its normal metabolic processes, produces waste which needs to be effectively disposed of. It's a fairly efficient operation, but there can be a lingering residue of harmful compounds. These undesirable chemicals and free radicals can be dangerous to body health; detoxifying or fasting is the best way to remove them.

I recommend detoxifying for 2-4 days, depending on your score / lifestyle. Be ready for some immediate bodily responses. By day two you may be experiencing some dizziness, so do be very careful when driving, exercising or using machinery. You may get headaches caused by a drop in blood sugar level, or by the absence of your normal tea or coffee fix. Day two might even see an increase in sweating, halitosis (bad breath) and a coated yellow tongue! But don't worry, there's no reason to panic: this is just the bacteria in the gut releasing chemicals which will then be absorbed by the stomach lining. If there are people giving you grief, making nasty comments about bad breath or yellow tongue, just tell them them to go back to their sausage rolls and cream cakes – or words to that effect! ☺

Nitro+ Diet Detox: daily diet routine

On rising (morning)

- A glass of warm water with lemon juice, which goes straight to the bowels and expels faecal matter from the day before. The temperature of the water is important, as cold water can shock and create wind in the tummy. This will remain part of your daily Nitro+ Diet routine.
- Fruit selection. Make your choice of two to three pieces of: watermelon, apples, pears, pineapples, cherries, peaches, apricots, berries, bananas.
- Two glasses (400 ml) of filtered water (distilled is even better, although only for a short period).

Mid morning

- 1 cup of herbal tea (dandelion, camomile, sage, peppermint, nettle), for liver detox
- 2 pieces of fruit from the list above
- 2 glasses of filtered water

Lunch

- 1 teaspoon of aloe vera oil (optional)
- Raw salad (tomato, pepper, spinach, lettuce, onion, kohlrabi, carrot, etc.)
- 500 ml of filtered water

Mid afternoon

- 1 or 2 cups of herbal tea of your choice
- 2 or 3 pieces of fruit of your choice

> ### *Dinner*
>
> * 1 teaspoon of aloe vera oil
> * Lightly steamed vegetables (steam no longer than 3 minutes) or raw salad, plus one cup of brown rice or pasta (alkaline)
> * 500 ml of filtered water with twist of lemon
>
> ### *After dinner*
>
> * Warm filtered water and lemon
> * One wild green-blue algae (optional)

Duration

How long you'll need to sustain this detox regime depends on how you scored in the twenty questions. For those of you with high scores, it will take four days to clear out all the toxins and tone and nourish the internal organs as mentioned above.

I would recommend detoxing like this for one day every season or quarter. That's only one day in 90, and only four days in a whole year. This will give your body time to cleanse and energize – your body is going to thank you for this in the long term. Look after your body: it's your greatest asset, one you should spend more time investing in than anything else.

Reactions

Be aware that this type of cleansing diet is going to have noticeable effects as it disrupts your normal consumption routine. Most people will experience symptoms of detoxifying by the end of day two, especially if having come off stimulants like tea or coffee. Energy levels may drop in the first 48 hours and you may get headaches or feel nausea. This is quite normal and is proof that your body needed cleansing. You can be confident that your energy levels will rapidly recover and your body will emerge feeling refreshed.

You'll have noticed that there's a lot of filtered water to be drunk throughout the day: this performs the essential detox task of flushing out your liver and kidneys.

Benefits

Apart from cleansing and nourishing your internal organs – pancreas, liver, kidneys, spleen, thyroid, adrenal glands, colon, and intestines – the Nitro+ Diet detox activation programme has a host of additional benefits. These include:

- Becoming aware of inappropriate eating habits
- Elimination of the burden of stimulants
- Expulsion of toxins
- Weight loss
- Clearer mental processes
- The body is re-vitalised and refreshed

This will prepare the body for the new fat burning environment we will start to build in Step 3 – eXchange.

Case Study # 3 – Steve

Just for a change, here's a male case study – Steve, aged 39. He had suffered from being overweight since he was a child, accumulating fat around the hips and abdominal area.

The Nitro+ Diet kicked off with a 5 day detox plan, which Steve found particularly hard, particularly the ban on caffeine. He followed a weight training regime three times a week, performing three sets using medium weights with a rep range of 10-12.

The results were pretty impressive:

Before Nitro+ training	
Start weight:	210 lbs
Body fat %-age:	30%
Lean mass:	147 lbs
Fat mass:	63 lbs
Category:	Overweight
After eight weeks	
Weight:	195 lbs
Body fat %-age:	22%
Lean mass:	152 lbs
Fat mass:	43 lbs
Category:	Above average

Over an eight week period the total weight lost was 15 pounds – just over a stone. The effect of weight training, which increases muscle mass and switches them into positive nitrogen balance, was clear. Body fat decreased by an amazing 8%; 20 lbs of body fat melted away, while muscle mass increased by 5 lbs.

Congratulations were definitely in order: Steve managed to achieve a major life-changing result by following the Nitro+ Diet and exercise plan.

Step 3–eXchange

Now that your body has had time to detoxify and cleanse it's time to create the perfect fat burning environment and eXchange your energy systems. The new system will help you lose a lot more body fat than any other traditional diet, without losing your muscle. Notice, it's all about losing body fat, not about weight loss.

The important thing to remember is, it's muscles that act as your fat burners – you wouldn't want to get rid of these! That would be like swapping a Mustang for a Metro: your engine just got downgraded, and your ability to burn energy would be drastically reduced.

Creating the right environment is very important. We've learned how to measure and calculate our daily protein, carbohydrates and fat. This is setting down a solid basis for our ideal fat burning environment. Next up, we'll need to pay close attention to insulin and blood glucose levels.

Step 3 will change the way you look, and quickly. This phase will shift your energy system from a dependence on external energy input to being able to source internal stored energy. Your fat burning switch will be turned on. When you've found out how to shift energy systems and toggle the fat burning switch you'll start to realise just how easy it is to burn off body fat – but you will need to learn how to ride the Insulin Rollercoaster.

Step on up for the insulin roller coaster

Roller coasters are not just for kids or theme park fanatics you know! Most of us go on this roller coaster on a daily basis without even knowing it. I've witnessed this roller coaster doing loop the loops up to 20 times per day! Yep, I'm serious, 20 times. It's thrills and spills galore, but not necessarily a whole lot of fun.

No wonder you feel giddy after eating the way you do. The sugary foods we like so much have a more or less instant impact on our body system, as blood glucose levels shoot up, followed closely by insulin peaking.

Our love affair with sugar is still the number one reason why we are getting fatter, and why obesity is such a global problem. It's easy to lay the blame on supermarkets, toying with our desires the way they do, offering us those tempting two for one deals on sugary snacks. Probe a bit deeper and you could lay your accusing finger on the corporations marketing this junk. But I'm hoping that you'll be able to turn that finger right around, and take personal responsibility for buying into this dangerous dependency.

Yep, it's time to exercise some self control. Next time you're in the supermarket, take a look at those shelves full of sweet temptation . . . and just walk on by. Be bold and resolute: you and your trolley are heading straight for the healthy eating zone.

Let's find out a little bit more about insulin and why we are getting fatter. Stay with me on this, because this information is going to be very useful.

The insulin and blood glucose see-saw

The energy we need to stay alive and functioning effectively comes from the food that we eat. It's our fuel, essentially. More precisely, and in common with most living organisms, we run on glucose. This is a compound of carbon, hydrogen and oxygen, which the body obtains from our food by breaking down carbohydrates such as starch.

Our bodies are able to store glucose, in the form of highly branched chains known as glycogen, but only to a limited extent. Mostly, glycogen is found in the liver (around 100 g, or up to 8% of the liver mass) or in the muscles (up to 500 g, representing 1-2% of overall muscle mass), plus there is a small amount circulating in the blood. Our glycogen levels determine how we look, whether we are lean or fat.

When we eat sugary or carbohydrate foods (remember, starch transforms to glucose) the pancreas reacts by releasing the hormone insulin into the bloodstream, in order to deal with the rising level of glucose. Too much glucose in the bloodstream is dangerous; insulin is able both to regulate the level as well as transform the glucose into useful energy. However, eating too much carbohydrate can lead to a parking problem, as the excess glycogen (surplus to our immediate energy needs) needs to be stored somewhere in the form of fat. Basically, after liver and muscles run out of room, it ends up parked up around our tummies, hips and thighs.

As insulin levels spike in response to high levels of glucose in the bloodstream, we experience a 'high', an insulin-induced exhilaration, followed inevitably by an energy crash which leaves us feeling tired and exhausted. This is the insulin roller coaster, a cycle of boom and bust on which we can appear to be trapped forever. It may sound like the stuff of nightmares, but there is a way to bring it safely to a halt.

Knowing how the body works is the key to stepping off the roller coaster. Understand that we have the power to regulate our insulin production, simply by keeping our sugar and carbohydrate intake at sensible levels. Once insulin levels subside and become more consistent the body will automatically switch energy systems from external – burning up glucose in the bloodstream – to internal – that is, converting stored fats into energy.

This is the secret, what the Nitro+ Diet is all about, switching from an external energy source to an internal one. When we consume large amounts of sugar or starch the internal energy system never gets a chance to kick in, and we end up just getting fatter and fatter. Our fat burner is switched off, fat storage on.

The consequences for our health can be serious – it's not just a matter of how we look. Too much glucose stashed away as fat during our insulin spikes can bring on type 2 diabetes, as well as leading to obesity.

Bread

Try to stay away from bread, particularly the highly processed sliced variety. It turns out that this is not so great after all. It's loaded with fast releasing carbohydrates, which will massively increase your blood glucose, sending insulin levels through the roof. If you want to help energize your body and strip away some body fat, just learn to say no.

Here's an interesting chart comparing various different types of breads, in terms of how the body reacts to the glucose input. High fibre rye bread clearly has least effect on blood sugar. Processed white bread, in contrast, generates a huge spike in glucose, followed by a significant and enduring trough. This is when you feel low energy, slumped out, and craving for more starchy carbohydrates to get back on top of the curve.

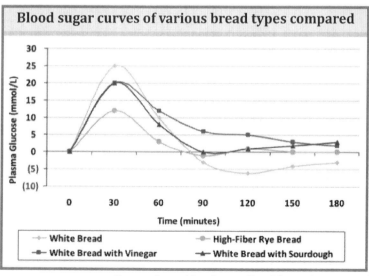

Source: http://pathways4health.org/resources/

So, is bread bad for us? It depends on what bread you are eating. White bread is made with highly refined flour and when consumed the carbohydrate is rapidly converted into glucose. White bread is a big NO-NO if you want to lose body fat.

According to a new study, just two or more daily servings of white bread can put you at a forty percent higher risk of becoming overweight and obese. Yep, you did read that right – a whopping 40%. The study monitored 9,267 Spanish graduate students over a five year period. No link was found to becoming overweight or obese amongst those who ate only whole grain bread.

Processed white bread has a very similar effect on the body as a can of fizzy pop – it sends glucose and insulin levels soaring. The resultant glycogen is stored away first in the muscles and liver, then, as fat, in all those familiar places – the spare tyres and muffin tops we carry around with us.

Going forward, I really recommend limiting the amount of bread you eat. If cutting out completely seems like too much to bear, go for the whole grain and sourdough breads.

Martinez-Gonzalez M, et al. European Congress on Obesity. 2014.

eXchanging energy systems

Gluconeogenesis

There is another way for the body to metabolise glucose from food. Gluconeogenesis is the metabolic process of making glucose from NON-carbohydrate foods such as protein. We all have this capability, but in most of us it never gets out of first gear, just trickling along. I'm going to tell you how to shift on up – this is going to make a big difference in burning off your body fat.

Eating more high quality protein, together with the right carbohydrates, will massively ramp up your gluconeo-genetic process. Your body will be able to tap into the glucogenic amino acids found in protein and other fuels. When we are consuming enough good quality protein we receive a full spectrum of amino acids, vital for production of such important agents as growth hormone, antibodies and haemoglobin.

The Nitro+ Diet is able to switch your energy systems from external to internal by lowering your glycogen reserves, tapping into the larger fat store for energy, and by exploiting the resources of non-carbohydrate foods such as protein.

Ketosis

Ketosis is something normally associated with diabetes or weight loss, but in itself it's not necessarily good or bad. A little more science will help us get a handle on this. So do bear with me – I'll try to make it easy to follow.

Ketosis is what happens in the body when it doesn't get enough carbohydrates to metabolise the glucose it needs for energy. It happens when we don't eat, limit our calories or starve ourselves on fad diets. It's just like a car running out of petrol – the dial hits the red zone and everything cranks to a halt. The body responds by burning up stored fat, producing in the process simple carbon compounds known as ketones.

This is quite different from gluconeogenesis and occurs when the carbohydrate intake is very low – less than 50 grams per day. When we are eating normally and not dieting our body does not normally produce or use ketones, although ketosis can occur during pregnancy, or after exercising, as demand for nutrients is increased. In these instances higher levels of ketones are found in the blood and are used for energy. Any ketones that are left over will be excreted via the kidneys and urine.

So, why should we worry about ketones? Well, there is a danger that excessive accumulation can result in the serious condition of ketoacidosis.

Ketosis blood concentration trigger levels

Blood concentration (millimolar)	Condition
<0.2	Not in ketosis
0.2-0.5	Slight/mild ketosis
0.5-3.0	Induced ketosis
2.5-3.5	Post exercise ketosis
3-6	Starvation ketosis
15-25	Ketoacidosis

Ketoacidosis

An excessive build up of ketones is known as ketoacidosis and is toxic to the body. Unregulated ketones can alter the chemical balance of the blood and if left untreated can prove fatal.

I don't want to be too much of a scaremonger here. Some research does suggest that ketogenic diets can help lower your risk of heart disease. Other studies show that specific very-low-carb diets can help people with metabolic syndrome, insulin resistance, and type 2 diabetes. To activate ketosis you need to be consuming less than 50 grams of carbohydrates per day. I would not recommend these type of diets, as that level of carbohydrates is far too low. The Nitro+ Diet allows for 50% of total calories from low glycaemic load carbohydrates. These parameters are much safer than the very low carbohydrate diets that are on the market and will not disrupt your normal lifestyle.

Things to avoid

Fizzy drinks

These might seem effervescent and fun, but actually they are exploding with disaster. The colourings used are carcinogenic. These drinks will weaken your bones, rot your teeth, cause stomach problems, make you irritable, play havoc with your insulin and blood glucose levels AND make you fat. The large quantities of sugar they contain will fill up your muscle and liver glycogen storage very quickly, and when this is full, the excess glucose is diverted by the liver to be stored as fat.

Now here's an amazing fact: if you substitute ordinary water for your daily bottle of fizzy pop, in just one year your body can lose up to 35 lbs – that's a whopping 2½ stone! How's that for an easy result! If you really can't do without that fizzy tingle on your tongue, go for carbonated water. It will feel just like the fizzy pop but without the souvenir muffin top.

Fruit Juice

It's a bit of a surprise to most people when I mention fruit juice being bad for you. It's not that it's bad in terms of the vitamins and minerals it contains, but it's the amount of sugar contained in fruit juice that's the problem – especially when you're trying to burn off body fat.

The sugar found in fruit is called fructose. In small amounts, as the delicious payoff to a piece of ripe fruit, there's nothing much to worry about; trouble only kicks in when all the pulp and fibre is removed, leaving only the concentrated fruit sugar. Fructose derived from corn syrup, the main sweetener in American soft drinks, is particularly problematic. Our bodies can only absorb about 25 grams of fructose at one time. Anything over this amount will go to the liver and be converted into fat.

Some people are fructose intolerant. This is when the body cannot absorb the excess fructose, leading to symptoms such as flatulence, cramps, bloating, belching and diarrhea or constipation.

How much sugar is in that drink?

Drink (8 fl.oz / 227 ml)	Calories	Total sugar (grams)
Sprite	100	26
Pepsi	100	28
Coca Cola classic	97	27
Gatorade G Cool Blue	50	14
Grape Juice	152	36
Pineapple Juice	132	25
Cranberry Juice	116	31
Apple Juice	114	24
Orange Juice	112	21

Source: U.S Dept. of Agriculture Nutrient Data Laboratory

This table compares the amounts of sugar typically contained in various fizzy drinks and fruit juices. It really is an eye opener! As you can see, in terms of sugar content there's not a lot to choose between them. In fact, it's best to cut out both fruit juices and fizzy drinks. Your insulin and blood glucose levels will stabilize, your energy levels will be more constant throughout the day and tiredness will be reduced. If you do feel thirsty, you need to rehydrate. Rather than go for the sugary drink, have some water – it will be kinder to your body and to your teeth and hydrate your body much more effectively.

Nitro+ Principle # 2
Avoid high sugar fruit juices, fizzy drinks & diet drinks

Diet drinks

I can hear you right now: "I don't drink the full sugar versions of these drinks. I drink the healthier diet or zero version." Well, I've got some important advice for you: STOP! These diet drinks disrupt your natural processes of appetite control and may result in consuming more food! It might seem like a good idea, but these drinks are really not good for you. Instead of sugar, they are loaded with chemical sweeteners that are potentially damaging to your health. You may well be consuming fewer calories but – weirdly – you'll end up with a bigger sugar craving than if you'd enjoyed the full sugar version. And, most likely, you'll make up for your 'abstinence' later in the day . . .

I see so many overweight or obese people drinking diet drinks, imagining they're doing themselves some good. It's tragic. Here's a question to stretch your brain cells. How many bottles of drink does the Coca Cola Corporation sell each day? 100 million? . . . 500 million? . . . 1 billion? . . . (not there yet?) . . . 1.5 billion? . . . actually, a stonking 1.8 BILLION bottles are sold by the Coca Cola company each and every day – and we wonder why we are getting fat !

Weight gain from diet drinks

A study was completed at the San Antonio Heart Study over a 7-8 year period monitoring weight changes in men and women. Amongst its results was the observation that weight gain and obesity was significantly higher amongst those drinking diet beverages. In another comparative study, monitoring adults over a two year period, it was shown that those consuming artificial sweetened drinks increased both their body fat and BMI.

Metabolic syndrome

This refers to a collection of conditions including high blood pressure and excess belly fat, which tend towards the onset of cardiovascular disease and diabetes. Recent studies demonstrate that the risk of developing this syndrome increases by as much as 200% in those consuming artificially sweetened (i.e. 'diet') drinks. You may think these diet drinks are doing some good for your muffin top, moobs and saddle bags – but it just ain't so.

Type 2 diabetes

In a recent European study the risk of developing type 2 diabetes was shown to double amongst those consuming diet drinks. Those people with a daily diet drink habit were particularly in danger. It might seem that I'm hammering hard on this point, but, hey, it's really just not worth it. Feeling thirsty? – go drink some water.

Hypertension and Cardiovascular Disease

The risk of developing coronary heart disease rises significantly for women consuming two or more artificially sweetened drinks per day. Two cups a day might not seem like much, but it really can make a big difference to your health. Ladies – stay away from the fizzy pop! Mineral water makes a lot more sense.

Nitro+ Principle # 3
Avoid Aspartame sweetener

Aspartame

Aspartame is one of the biggest rogues on the food additive market. It's the technical name for artificial sweetener brands such as NutraSweet, Equal and Equal-Measure, available in little micro-pills that can be as much as one hundred times sweeter than sugar. Avoid it at all costs. It's been used in carbonated beverages since 1983, ironically as the healthy sugar-free option. Actually, it's responsible for around 75% of all adverse reactions to food additives. It's astonishing that this stuff has been approved for human consumption.

Some of the symptoms of ingesting Aspartame are:

- Weight gain
- Dizziness
- Headaches
- Fatigue
- Muscle spasms
- Seizures
- Joint pain
- Heart palpitations

And it doesn't stop there . . . the chronic illnesses listed below can be worsened by consuming aspartame.

- Multiple sclerosis
- Epilepsy
- Parkinson's
- Diabetes
- Brain tumours
- Birth defects
- Chronic fatigue syndrome

As you can see, this stuff really is dangerous, something you should be steering well clear of. Check the label on all of the low diet, low sugar drinks and you will be surprised. Don't buy the low sugar, or 'sugar-free' versions of anything – they are just removing the sugar and putting in these dreadful, harmful chemicals. You'd actually be better off with the sugar, as these chemicals will cause havoc in your body and you'll end up putting on more weight in the long run.

Well, it's a big problem that's not going away any time soon. The artificial sweetener market is a huge multi-billion dollar industry . . . enough said.

Mercola.com

Nitro+ Principle # 4
Avoid Starchy Foods

These foods are also very good at filling up your glycogen storage. Try to move away from relying on high starch foods such as potatoes, rice, pasta and breads. Consuming a big plateful of any of these foods at one sitting is a sure way to get fat, just as much as drinking fizzy drinks and fruit juices. These types of food convert to glucose very quickly, pressing the starter button on the insulin roller coaster. Remember, the more insulin our body produces, the more fat is shunted off into fat storage.

For years we've been told to obtain a third of our food from these high carbohydrate sources. Maybe that made some sort of sense in the post-war austerity years, when a small amount of high quality protein was a real under-the-counter luxury, but it's not a way to lose body fat built up in times of abundance. Avoid these starchy foods and keep your intake of saturated fats under control and you'll be surprised how quickly the fat starts to fall off.

I could go into a lot more detail about starchy food . . . but maybe that's for another book!

Creating the fat burning environment

It's actually not that hard to create the perfect fat burning environment – it just takes a bit of willpower, determination and discipline, together with a clear sense of direction. I'm here to help provide some guidance. There's an easy-to-follow plan, plus I've put together a list of my Top Ten foods that are low in glycaemic load, low in carbohydrates, and high in protein and fibre. At the end of this book (Appendix A) there'll also be some useful recipes to give you some menu-planning inspiration.

Why is lemon juice so important?

Remember how often lemon juice showed up in the detox diet? I promised then that it would also play a significant role in your Nitro+ Diet. It's time to find out why.

After you've brushed your teeth, warm water with fresh lemon juice is the best way to start your day. Here are five very good reasons:

1. It cleanses your system. Lemon juice make you want to pee. Toxins are therefore released more rapidly from the body while the citric acid wakes up the liver, aids detoxification and maximizes enzyme function.
2. It boosts immunity, by virtue of the high levels of vitamin C contained in lemons. They are also high in potassium, great for controlling blood pressure and inflammation.
3. It clears the skin: lemon juice can fight the ageing process and reduce wrinkles and fine lines.

4. It aids digestion. Shortly after drinking your lemon juice you may feel the need to go to the toilet. Lemon juice flushes out unwanted toxins and materials from the body. It also kickstarts the liver into producing bile, an acid essential for digestion.

5. It aids weight loss. Yep, it also encourages weight loss by fighting hunger cravings. Studies have shown that people who consume more alkaline than acidic foods lose weight faster.

How to prepare your lemon juice

It's best if you can use purified or filtered water. If this isn't available, then freshly boiled water that has cooled is fine. Avoid boiling or ice-cold water as both these can create unwanted wind and use valuable energy in bringing them to body temperature. Always try to use fresh lemons, preferably organic.

Okay, now here comes the technical bit: squeeze half of the lemon into the warm water and drink it down. Do this every day before doing anything, preferably 10 minutes before your high protein breakfast. For added variety, you could add some freshly grated ginger or crank it up with a little cayenne.

Tasty yummies.com

Nitro+ Principle # 5
Drink warm water with fresh lemon juice upon rising, before breakfast

Next up is some guidance for your daily diet regime. Please note that the percentages given for proteins and carbohydrates refer to your daily allowance of these food types, rather than the proportional composition of the meals in question.

Zero carb, high protein breakfast

20% Protein, 0% Carbohydrates

Once you have been cleansed and refreshed from the lemon juice it's time to stoke yourself up for the day, firing up your fat burning engines. At breakfast you need to make sure the proteins are high and the carbohydrates as close to zero as possible. So, no toast! You are aiming to consume around 20% of your daily protein intake at breakfast-time, so if you need 100 grams of protein per day, 20 grams should be for breakfast.

Select items from my Top Ten protein foods. Eggs are always easy first thing in the morning and ready in a matter of minutes. My personal favourite is scrambled. It's good quality protein, and if you want to reduce the fat to cholesterol quotient, just remove one or two yolks before you start. Whisk them up, pop them in the micro-wave, every 30 seconds scramble them up with a fork and – hey presto – you'll have perfect scrambled eggs in two minutes, high in protein and easy to prepare.

One of the big problems I've noticed with people who are overweight or obese is that they don't eat breakfast. Remember, breakfast is literally about breaking the fast after sleeping. When we eat breakfast it wakes up the body's digestive system, kicking it into gear, setting it about generating and distributing the energy you'll need for the day. Your fat burning switch will be turned on, creating a positive nitrogen balance in your muscles.

Those who eat a good breakfast tend to eat less for lunch and dinner and also be less tempted to snack during the day. Protein foods are also slow to digest, so you stay feeling full for longer. So, don't skip breakfast and consume good quality proteins.

Mid-morning break (around 10-11am)

15% daily carbohydrate allowance, 10% protein

Select some items from the fruits and snack charts. Aim to consume 15% of your carbohydrate allowance when snacking: for example, if you need to consume 180 grams of carbohydrates per day, aim to consume around 18 grams of carbohydrates mid-morning, together with a small amount of protein. I recommend a small serving of low glycaemic fruits, such as 8 strawberries, a couple of plums, or half a grapefruit. For the protein, a handful of nuts would be ideal.

Lunch

35% of your carbohydrates (including 10 g of fibre), 35% protein

This is going to be your largest meal of the day. It makes sense to consume most of your calories at lunch as you'll have all afternoon to burn them off. Recent research has demonstrated that the body's ability to make use of the sugar in food fluctuates throughout the day in harmony with your body clock.

You will be consuming 35% of your carbohydrates at lunch, plus 35% of your protein, with around 10 grams of fibre included in your carbohydrates.

Some tasty lunch recommendations are:

- Grilled chicken with lentil and black bean salad
- 3-4 egg omelette with bean salad and couscous
- Halibut and sweet potato with salad
- Grilled cod with sweet potato

Again, don't forget to drink plenty of fluids – AFTER, not during, your lunch.

> ### *Nitro+ Principle # 6*
> ## Lunch like a prince and dine like a pauper

Mid-afternoon snack (3-4 pm)

15% carbohydrates 10% protein

Your mid-afternoon snack is more or less the same as your elevenses. Check out the fruits and snacks chart for an appropriate selection of fruit, nuts or seeds.

Dinner (before 8 pm)

Consume 35% of your low glycaemic load carbohydrates here and 25% of your protein.

This meal is going to be significantly smaller than your lunch serving. Try to eat your dinner before it gets too late, ideally between 6.00 and 7.30. This will give your body time in the evening to digest the food and you'll end up sleeping a lot better. If you eat late, especially fatty foods, you're bound to put on fat, as the body simply stores away its surplus nutrients. Also, your digestive system doesn't get a chance to shut down, keeping you awake with its churning and gurgling.

My Top Ten low GL carbohydrate foods

Food	How much?	Carbs (g)	Protein (g)	Fat (g)	Fibre (g)	Sodium (mg)	GL
Lettuce	100 g	2.9	1.4	0.2	1.3	28	<15
Spinach	100 g	3.6	2.9	0.4	2.2	79	<15
Cucumber	100 g	3.6	0.6	0.1	0.5	2	<15
Mushrooms	5 medium	3	3	0	1	15	<15
Asparagus	100 g	3	2	0	<1	0	<15
Yam	100 g	28	1.5	0.2	4.1	9	9
Wholemeal spaghetti	100 g	27	5	1	5	3	9
Sweet potato	100 g	20	1.6	0	3	55	11
Couscous	100 g	23	3.8	0.8	1.4	5	16
Pumpernickel bread	2 slices	24	4.6	6.2	3.4	310	17

My Top Ten low GL, high protein and fibre foods (vegetarian option)

Food	How much?	Carbs (g)	Protein (g)	Fat (g)	Fibre (g)	Sodium (mg)	GL
Split peas	100 g	21	8	0.4	8	2	4
Lentils	100 g	20	9	0.4	8	2	4
Black beans	100 g	20	9	1	9	1	9
Lima beans (frozen)	100 g	20	8	0.4	7	2	7
Artichokes	1 medium	11	3.3	0.2	5	94	3
Peas	100 g	5	5	0.4	5	5	2
Broccoli	100 g	8	4	3	3	80	<15
Brussels sprouts	100 g	7	3	0	3	21	<15
Sun dried tomatoes	100 g	56	14	3	12	247	22
Quinoa	100 g	21	4	2	3	7	10

My Top Ten Protein Foods

Food	How much?	Carbs (g)	Protein (g)	Fat (g)	AAD*	BV*	GL*
Whey protein (powder)	30 g	3.2	21.5	1.5	1	159	<15
Whole egg	1 large	0.6	6	5	1	100	<15
Halibut	½ fillet	0	36	2.6	1	80	<15
Tuna (skipjack)	½ fillet	0	44	2	61	83	<15
Cod	½ fillet	0	20	1.6	0.96	82	<15
Salmon (unsmoked)	½ fillet	0	40	27			<15
Chicken breast (cooked)	100 g	0	25	13	1	79	<15
Turkey breast (cooked)	100 g	0	29	7	0.97	79	<15
Cottage cheese	100 g	3.4	11	4.3	1	79	<15
Quorn (mince)	100 g	9	11	3	0.99		<15

*AAD: Amino acid digestibility

*BV: Biological Value

*GL: Glycaemic Load

My Top Ten Fruits

Food	How much?	Carbs (g)	Protein (g)	Fat (g)	Fibre (g)	Sodium (mg)	GL
Strawberries	8 medium	11	1	0	2	8	4
Apricot	1 medium	4	0.5	0.1	0.7	3	10
Grapefruit	Half	15	1	0	2	11	6
Plum	1 medium	8	0.5	0.2	0.9	7	7
Kiwi Fruit	2 medium	20	1	1	4	13	6
Peach	1 medium	15	1	0.5	2	13	7
Sweet cherries	100 g	12	1	0.3	1.6	8	8
Canteloupe melon	Quarter	12	1	0	1	11	4
Watermelon	1 wedge (1/6)	12	1.7	0.4	1.1	18	7
Blueberries	120 g	30	1	0	19	19	15

My Top Ten low GL drinks /beverages

Drink	How much?	Carbs (g)	Protein (g)	Fat (g)	Fibre (g)	Sugar (g)	GL
Water bottled /tap	180 ml	0	0	0	0	0	0
Green tea (no sugar)	180 ml	0	0	0	0	0	0
Black coffee (no sugar)	180 ml	0	0.3	0	0	0	0
Soy milk	180 ml	15	8	4.2	1.5	124	8
Tomato juice	180 ml	8	1.4	0.1	0.7	18	6
Grapefruit juice (unsweetened)	180 ml	22.7	1.24	0.25	0.2	2	8
Apple juice (unsweetened)	180 ml	29	0.1	0.3	0.2	7	7
Carrot juice	180 ml	16.4	1.7	0.27	1.4	51	7
Orange juice (unsweetened)	180 ml	18.3	0.7	0.2	0.2	8	13
Banana /soymilk smoothie	180 ml	16	5.3	2.7	2.7	6	5

My Top Ten Snacks

Food	How much?	Carbs (g)	Protein (g)	Fat (g)	Fibre (g)	Salt (mg)	GL
Almonds	100 g	22	21	49	12	1	<15
Hazelnuts	100 g	17	15	61	10	0	<15
Macademia	100 g	14	8	76	9	5	<15
Pecan	100 g	14	9	72	10	0	<15
Walnuts	100 g	14	15	65	7	2	<15
Tofu	100 g	1.9	8	4.8	0.3	28	<15
Peanuts	100 g	16	26	49	8	18	<15
Cashews	100 g	33	15	46	3	16	<15
Pistachios	100 g	28	20	45	10	1	<15
Brazil nuts	100 g	12	14	66	8	3	<15

Source: International Table of Glycaemic Index and Load

Summary:

How to create the perfect fat burning environment

- Cut out fast food
- Cut out fizzy drinks, diet drinks and limit fruit juices
- Cut down on the sugar, tea, coffee (black is ok), cigarettes and alcohol
- Eat more protein with low GL foods
- Drink warm water with lemon juice upon rising
- Lunch like a prince and dine like a pauper
- Consume low GL carbohydrates with protein

The Cup, the Saucepan and the Bath

Imagine a bath. Inside the bath is a medium sized saucepan and a cup. In this case the bath, metaphorically speaking, is your body's total fat storage capacity, the cup is liver storage and the saucepan is muscle storage. When we eat carbohydrates, especially refined high sugar carbohydrates, glucose enters into the blood and, in response, insulin is released to manage the blood glucose level. Glycogen is produced; where is it going to go?

Well, first of all (in terms of our analogy) it goes into the cup (i.e. the liver), then into the saucepan (muscle) and when both these are full it starts spilling over into the bath. The bath – our surplus fat storage – keeps on filling up. Maybe at first you don't notice, but sure enough, the water level gets deeper and deeper. There's sure to be trouble on the way . . .

Now, when we drink fizzy drinks, fruit juices and tuck into chocolate and cakes, we fill up the cup and saucepan pretty quickly. We then have a meal and, because the liver and muscle storage is maxed out, the resulting glycogen is diverted into the large fat storage. Cup and saucepan are already full, so the bath starts filling up.

Try to remember this analogy and it will serve you well in the future. By following the Nitro+ Diet you will no longer be dumping loads of excess glucose into the blood-stream and cranking up the insulin roller coaster. Gaps and pockets in the muscles will be created, allowing some of the blood glucose to be used for replenishment rather than being stashed away. Avoiding or reducing sugary, high carbohydrate foods will reduce insulin levels and set your fat burning switch to On.

Here's another way to think of fat storage, in terms of digital memory.

Gigabytes, capacity and fat storage

When we are looking to buy phones, music players, computers and even TVs we are always looking for a device with plenty of digital memory – storage, essentially. As the technology has developed, storage has got larger – much larger – while the devices have got ever smaller. Without sufficient storage we wouldn't be able to download films, music or take loads of pointless selfies. Let's use this way of thinking to help us understand how the body is able to accumulate so much fat.

Muscle storage:160 GB (300 - 500 g of glycogen)

Remember how we talked about glycogen storage earlier? Glycogen, the product of insulin and glucose interaction, is first of all stored in the muscles, with a smaller amount circulating in the blood stream. However, this muscle glycogen storage is strictly limited; eating lots of high carbohydrate foods will rapidly exhaust its carrying capacity.

The muscles can hold around 300-500 grams of glycogen, which amounts to around 1400-2000 calories, capable of powering you through around 80-100 minutes of endurance exercise, depending on intensity. This is why athletes need to stay well hydrated so as to keep their glycogen stores topped up. Watch the tennis players at Wimbledon, see how they are constantly re-hydrating and consuming gels and high sugar isotonic drinks to maintain their energy levels. A reduction in muscle glycogen will be sure to affect their performance. Muscle glycogen is used locally by the active muscles and can be quickly replaced by consuming simple carbohydrates.

Liver storage: 40 GB (100 grams of glycogen)

The liver is a much more complex organ. Liver storage is very similar to the muscle glycogen storage but has a smaller storage capacity than the muscles. The liver is capable of holding around 100 grams of glycogen, equiv-alent to 400 calories.

Fat storage – unlimited

At least you know where you stand with digital memory; there's a maximum capacity, just like there's a definitive size to your metaphorical bath. With the human body it's not possible to be so specific – I don't know why God designed us like this but . . . fact is, our fat storage is . . . wait for it . . . unlimited!

Once our muscle and liver storage is full, the glycogen is metabolised into triglyceride fat and packed away. I think you know where it goes! Triglycerides can be broken down into fatty acids by the body when it needs to use it as an energy source, but otherwise this fat just keeps on building up. Our body's unlimited storage capability has the potential to supply us with well in excess of 100,000 calories. Which sounds like an unnecessarily large amount of fuel supply to be sloshing around in the tank.

By now you should be starting to understand how we can so easily pile on the pounds and pack on the lard.

How we burn fuel

All fuels burn at a different rate. It's no different with the various categories of foodstuff we rely on to provide us with energy. This is a consequence of the varying proportions of carbon, hydrogen and oxygen atoms in fats, proteins, and carbohydrates. They have different energy densities, which affects how readily they are absorbed, and how quickly they can be converted into energy.

Carbohydrates are the body's favourite source of fuel. They offer easily accessible energy, in the form of muscle glycogen and blood glucose. When we exercise the primary fuel is adenosine triphosphate (ATP), which is formed a lot more readily from carbohydrates than from fat.

One big problem with traditional diets is that, in reducing calorific intake, they strip away valuable muscle tissue along with some of the surplus fat. When the diet is over the body is left feeling robbed of its nutrients, so it activates the survival switch. It starts demanding more carbs, inevitably piling up more fat than ever. What's going on here? Fat – stored energy – is your backup reserve. Your survival switch gets activated to make sure there's enough in the storehouse, just in case starvation – the sense of being deprived of essential nutrients – kicks in again. There's not much we can do about this, it's just the way we have evolved.

Aerobic Exercise

Aerobic exercise is the sort of short duration, low intensity workout we can undertake without drawing upon the body's deeper stores of energy.

It's fuelled by adenosine triphosphate (ATP), derived principally from carbohydrates. Carbohydrates are formed into ATP twice as much as fats. Yep, you read that right – carbs are the body`s number one fuel when doing aerobic exercise – not fat but carbohydrates.

Anaerobic Exercise

So how is anaerobic exercise different? The body can only go so far on the energy resources held, in the form of blood glucose and glycogen, in the bloodstream and muscles. Increased levels of exertion demand a different sourcing strategy, digging deeper into the body's box of metabolic tricks.

Amazingly, when we are in the anaerobic zone carbohydrates are formed into ATP five times as much as fats – that's a 5 fold (500%) increase! Fat is really not much good as a fuel when completing anaerobic exercise.

Utilisation

So, how much nourishment can the body absorb at one time? Knowing this is going to be a big help as you set about planning your meals for the Nitro+ Diet. If we eat too much, or the wrong sort of food, we're going to get fat.

It comes back to the good old saying: everything in moderation!

Maximum Protein Absorption

There are reports that you can only absorb between five and nine grams of protein per hour, and the rest of the protein you eat will be used for energy or turned into fat. Additionally, there is a limit to how much protein you can absorb in one day, according to an article on the University of California, LA, website, which notes that the maximum usable amount of protein is 0.91 grams per pound of body weight per day. This means that someone weighing 150 pounds won't be able to process more than 136 grams of protein per day, even if this protein is spread out in multiple servings throughout the day. Not to worry! This is well above the recommended dietary allowance for protein of 46 grams per day for women and 56 grams per day for men. It's best to spread out your protein intake throughout the day, across breakfast, lunch and dinner.

Not all fat is bad

You may have noticed I haven't been talking much about fat, but that's not because fat isn't important. We all need fats; they play a major role in our metabolism. And it will really pay to know what sort of fats are particularly good for us, and which it would be best to avoid.

Many people think all fat is bad, but it has played a crucial role in human development. Way back in prehistory, when folks were hanging out in caves, keeping a watchful eye out for passing mammoths and sharpening their flint axes in readiness for the hunt, red meat came to feature more regularly in their diets. This red meat was high in protein and fats – saturated fats. This increased amount of animal fat allowed the brain, over time, to develop. We got smarter . . . started to put two and two together . . . to evolve – and the rest is history!

Fats, also known as triglycerides, are compounds of fatty acids and the alcohol glycerol. They are all composed of carbon and hydrogen in various configurations, giving the different types of fat their individual characteristics – for example, unsaturated fats have one or more double bonded carbons in their molecular chain, whereas saturated fats have none of these double bonds.

All fats contain more calories than proteins and carbohydrates, roughly 9 calories per gram compared to four in both protein and carbohydrates. That's more than double the calorific content, so you can appreciate that high fat diets are very likely to make you fat and are not recommended for your health – unless you happen to be an Eskimo!

Let's take a look at the three main categories of fat. I have made this as easy to understand as possible so that it's practical and useful for you.

Good fats

Polyunsaturated fats

These fats are good for your heart, and much better for you overall than saturated fat. Try to replace saturated fat with polyunsaturated fat. At room temperature polyunsaturated fats are typically liquid, but start to turn solid when chilled.

Examples of polyunsaturated fat include:

- Fish (e.g. salmon, mackerel, tuna, herring)
- Soybean oil
- Sunflower oil
- Walnuts
- Flax seeds
- Corn oil

Benefits

Polyunsaturated fats have some fantastic health benefits. They can help lower levels of bad cholesterol, also known as low density lipoprotein (LDL). This cholesterol is notoriously 'sticky', tending to attach itself to blood vessel walls, leading to increased blood pressure and heightened risk of strokes and heart attacks.

Polyunsaturated fats also contain the very important omega 3 and omega 6 fats, which play a key role in brain function and cell growth, clotting and muscle movement.

Mono-unsaturated fats

These fats have a single carbon-to-carbon double bond and have two fewer hydrogen molecules than saturated fats. Like polyunsaturates they tend to be liquid at room temperature.

Foods high in this fat include:

- Peanuts
- Avocados
- Nuts
- Olive oil
- Canola (rape or safflower)

Mono-unsaturated fats are also good for your heart. Just take a look at the Mediterranean diet. It's naturally high in mono-unsaturated fats, thanks to the ever-present olive oil. Drizzled over salads, or as a principal constituent of dips, it's an indispensable staple. Not only is it so much healthier than butter or margarine, but it's simple to use – just splash it on! Next time you're in your local Italian restaurant feel free to take special pleasure in helping yourself to the olive oil and balsamic vinegar that are sure to be on the table.

Bad Fats

Trans fat ('hydrogenated vegetable fat')

This fat is the worst type of dietary fat and should be avoided at all costs. It is the product of an industrial process known as hydrogenation, by which liquid oil is made to set solid. It's been widely employed by the food industry, very often in conjunction with palm oil, allowing baked goods to be kept for an extremely long time. It is, however, a terrible health risk.

Hydrogenated fat increases levels of bad cholesterol (LDL), and provokes systemic inflammation which may lead to strokes, diabetes, and coronary heart disease. Research from the Harvard School of Public Health has found that even small amounts of trans-fats can be harmful. A daily intake of just 2% trans fat can increase your risk of heart disease by an alarming 23%! This stuff is bad, very bad. Stay away from fast food and convenience food in supermarkets, because the manufacturers of these items really haven't got the message. Check on the back of the label . . . if it contains hydrogenated fats, shun it like the plague.

Saturated fats

Saturated fats are another one to steer clear of. Its bad guy status is more well known than trans fat, and most people already know to keep this out of their shopping trolley. It's good to see how people are increasingly paying attention to the ingredients list on the back of the packet, and that these have been made easier to decipher.

Like you'd expect, these fats are saturated – with hydrogen. There are no double carbon bonds linking the atoms. Saturated fat has long been associated with increased risk of heart disease, stroke, and even cancer. It's clearly a good idea to reduce the amount of saturated fats in your diet.

Various foods contain saturated fats as part of their fatty mix. High proportions are found in the following foods:

- Red meat
- Coconut oil
- Cheese, butter & cream
- Whole Milk
- Baked goods

Harvard Health publications: *The truth about fats: the good, the bad, and the in-between*

Nitro+ Principle # 7
Stick to polyunsaturated and mono-unsaturated fats

Coming up, here's another Top Ten, though really these belong on the Bottom!

Top Ten Saturated Fat Foods: to avoid

Food	Saturated fat per 100g
Hydrogenated oils (palm oil)	93.7 g
Coconut (desiccated)	57.2 g
Animal fats	52.3 g
Butter	51.4 g
Chocolate (baking chocolate)	32.4 g
Fish oils (sardines)	29.9 g
Goat cheese	24.6 g
Cream	23.0 g
Nuts	15.1 g
Processed meats	14.9 g

USDA National Nutrient Database for Standard Reference, Release 26-27

Stay positively balanced with high nitrogen foods

> ### *Nitro+ Principle # 8*
> ## Eat a protein only breakfast

Why is this so important? Well, just take a minute to consider your normal morning routine. Maybe, like a lot of people with a busy lifestyle, there's no time to waste. It's get up, brush teeth, quick shower, maybe a quick coffee with toast, and off they go out the door. If they're trying to be health conscious, maybe they'll be pouring so-called 'healthy' cereals into their bowl. But . . . wait a minute, just how much sugar is in that crunchy concoction?

When we wake up in the morning our bodies, starved overnight and in a muscle wasting catabolic state, are craving our most preferred source of energy – carbohydrates. The overnight gluconeogenetic metabolic state will be able to switch back into glycolysis in the aftermath of a carbohydrate-rich breakfast. But from the point of view of the Nitro+ Diet, that's not such a good idea.

To create an anabolic fat burning environment, you should consume lots of protein at breakfast. Stay well away from sugars and carbohydrates as these will boost your blood sugar levels and create an unwanted insulin spike followed by unnecessary fat storage. This might take a bit of growing accustomed to, but just like any habit, you will get used to it.

Consuming protein at breakfast provides a greater feeling of fullness and less craving for elevenses snacks followed by a large lunch. Consuming carbohydrates at breakfast, on the other hand, has a dampening effect on the fat burning enzymes acquired while sleeping and stimulates the production of fat accumulating enzymes.

This is a very important fact to remember. Of all the things you read in this book, do try and hang on to these key principles: ***no carbs after 8pm in the evening and consume a protein only breakfast.*** This will create a more efficient fat burning environment and strip away fat like you wouldn't believe. Don't just take my word for it, try this principle for just one week and you will notice the difference. Not just the way your body looks in the mirror, but your whole body metabolism is going to change. It will be a major turning point in your life.

A study was carried out at the University of Missouri amongst three groups of obese or overweight people, comparing the effects of a normal cereal breakfast, a high protein egg and pork breakfast and no breakfast at all. How satiated did each group feel? The group that consumed the high protein egg and pork breakfast experienced a very clear decrease in hunger together with a heightened feeling of fullness compared to the other groups. Moreover, it was found that those who skipped breakfast entirely showed significant increases in body fat mass by comparison to the other higher protein groups.

Protein Supplement

To help you understand why protein makes such an

effective breakfast, I'd like to introduce you to a measure known as Thermic Effect of Food, or TEF. This relates to the amount of energy, relative to the resting metabolic rate, needed to process and store the food that we eat. Different types of food have a different TEF, and the TEF of protein is particularly advantageous.

For protein the TEF is around 25%, whereas for carbohydrates and fats it can be as low as 5%. This means that, simply in the process of digesting and storing your breakfast fuel, you'll be using up a comparatively greater number of calories – and that means less fat!

If you're wondering if there's an easy way to load up on breakfast protein (faster even than the scrambled eggs I mentioned earlier!), then whey and casein protein powder could be the solution. Consuming a 20-25 gram serving for breakfast would definitely help set up your fat loss environment. Now, I know protein powders have had a bad press over years, but they do serve a purpose. They are very simple and easy to use, allowing you to get good quality proteins into your system with the minimum of fuss.

Whey protein will give you the quick boost of amino acids and the casein will slowly release energy all the way through to lunchtime. Casein and whey protein are also fantastic in the evening as they contain high levels of the amino acids leucine and glutamine. These have been proven to keep your muscles in the positive nitrogen balance environment.

Of course, if you do have enough time in the morning to prepare something a little more elaborate, why not go for eggs or fish, with a glass of milk for the slow releasing casein. Make sure it's quality protein, with a high biological value. Don't underestimate vegetable protein!

Whey and Casein compared

Whey and casein are different types of protein, both present in milk. Here's a table indicating some of their significant differences.

	Whey	Casein
Complete protein?	Yes	Yes
High in leucine?	Yes	No
High in glutamine?	No	Yes
Absorption rate?	Fast	Slow
Duration of elevated blood amino acids?	Short	Long

Why Casein is important

Casein is the most abundant protein in milk. In water it is relatively insoluble, but in milk it is suspended in particles known as casein micelles. There are many good reasons why I recommend casein protein as part of your Nitro+ Diet.

Retains muscle

Casein protein is a powerhouse when it comes to fat loss. It digests relatively slowly and provides the body with a sustained release of amino acids for as long as eight hours. It is naturally high in glutamine (often known as

L-glutamine). Glutamine can be converted to glucose in the kidneys and can divert the glucose away from fat storage and utilised for energy. On its own, studies have shown that supplementation with glutamine resulted in a loss of bodyfat and a reduction in cravings for alcohol and sugar.

One study was conducted in Boston, comparing the effects of casein protein hydrolysate and whey protein hydrolysate, in terms of lean muscle mass gains and total fat loss. Two separate groups consumed either one or the other, whilst both also eating a lower carbohydrate diet and doing some weight training.

While both groups did show fat loss, the group using the casein protein showed greater mean fat loss and higher increases in strength for the chest, shoulders and legs.

The casein group came out of the study with a higher lean mass, which points towards casein being fantastic at creating a positive nitrogen balance in muscle tissue and, therefore, at maintaining muscle. This is mainly due to the high levels of glutamine, the most abundant amino acid in muscle tissue. Muscle glutamine levels drop very rapidly when we are training and catabolism sets in. Consuming a protein supplement after training allows the muscles to shift from catabolic to anabolic, thanks largely to the glutamine boost. Glutamine is also important for:

- Protein synthesis (just as any other of the 20 protein-ogenic amino acids)
- Cellular energy, as a source, next to glucose

- Anabolic processes and maintaining positive nitrogen balance.

Contains lots of calcium

The high levels of calcium in casein protein are a definite benefit when it comes to total fat loss.

I have heard several times in the press that dairy products can make you fat and slow you down. This is complete and utter nonsense. Let me tell you about a study conducted by the International Journal of Obesity. They observed that those participants who, over the course of 24 hours, combined a high calcium intake with a normal protein intake showed increased faecal fat and energy excretion for that day of approximately 350 kJ more than those who either took in a low calcium, normal protein intake or those who consumed a high protein, high calcium intake. That's right – casein protein will help create a positive nitrogen retention in your muscles and, thanks to its calcium component, is capable of out-performing a very high protein diet!

Casein can also help promote colon health.

To summarize, I would recommend consuming casein protein powders in the evening so that you get a slow release of protein when you are sleeping and then also again in the morning for a sustained release of amino acids. This will create a fat burning zone and allow you switch your muscles from catabolic to anabolic and turbo-charge your fat burners!

Remember, with the Nitro+ Diet the aim is to keep the muscle, burn the fat!

Switching from catabolic to anabolic

To enable the switch from catabolic to anabolic I would recommend a protein supplement that contains both casein and whey proteins. This will provide high levels of the amino acids leucine and glutamine, both of which play a significant role in creating and encouraging a positive nitrogen balance environment. Remember, this is the environment which will preserve your invaluable muscle tissue. Toned skeletal muscle is your key to burning body fat.

The window of opportunity

Are you listening carefully? Here's a little secret that can make a big difference in how you look.

There are special times in every week when, if you know what you are about, you can surge ahead with your muscle development and your fat loss programme. These windows of opportunity will enable your body to increase nutrient uptake by 400%. Yep, that's 400% – FOUR FOLD! So where can you find these windows?

Every time you exercise, go out for a run, or train with weights your muscles become much more receptive to nutrients; in effect, they turn into large sponges, desperate to soak up extra fuel. So when is this special window? It's within ONE HOUR of finishing your training. Yep, it's that easy. Straight after your training, help yourself to one serving of carbohydrates washed down with 20-25 grams of protein. This is where protein supplements really come in handy. Not only are they convenient, but they are packed with the top quality proteins and amino acids your muscles are crying out for. Just make sure that your protein supplement has the full spectrum of essential amino acids.

By following this simple principle you will allow your muscles to recover faster, turning off the catabolic muscle wasting switch and activating your fat burners.

There you go – I've shared my big secret! It's something that has made a big difference for me. I'm still amazed how effective it is. It's so simple . . . do give it a go . . . you won't be disappointed.

> ### Nitro+ Principle # 9
> **Consume protein within one hour of finishing training, together with some simple carbohydrates for anti-catabolism**

Amino Acids

This is really a journey of discovery! Amino acids – what do they do? They're actually quite important for our task in hand: basically, they are the building blocks of muscle-building protein. We can divide amino acids into two groups: essential and non essential.

Essential amino acids

These are amino acids which are vital for your health, but which the body is unable to synthesize through metabolic process. They must be supplied by the protein we consume. They include:

- Isoleucine
- Leucine
- Lysine
- Methionine,
- Phenylalanine
- Threonine
- Tryptophan
- Valise

Non-essential amino acids

Don't be fooled be the name. We definitely need these too, but the body is capable of manufacturing them using its clever metabolic toolkit – so they don't need to be a part of your diet. They include:

- Glutamine
- Arginine
- Proline
- Serine
- Glutamate
- Alanine
- Tyrosine
- Cysteine
- Aspartate
- Glycine
- Taurine

Did you ever make cottage cheese? Whey is the liquid which remains after you've precipitated the solids out of milk. It contains quite a bit of protein (about 10% of the total dry solids in whey): the total protein in milk is 20% whey, 80% casein. Whey protein is an important source of amino acids, particularly when fortified with an essential amino acid mix.

A study was carried out on older obese adults by Robert Coker, PhD, an associate professor of geriatrics at the University of Arkansas for Medical Sciences, Little Rock. The study compared two types of meal replacements. One was a whey protein replacement without essential amino acids. The other was a whey meal replacement with essential amino acids. Both groups lost 7% of their total body weight, but body fat loss was distinctly higher amongst the group consuming the extra amino acids.

So that's why some amino acids are essential. Don't underestimate this: consume essential amino acids with your protein replacement and you will burn off more body fat – it's as simple as that.

www.nutritionj.com/content/11/1/105/abstract

Nitro+ Principle # 10
Snack between meals on fruit, nuts and seeds

Reducing your carbohydrate intake and cranking up your protein is quite likely to leave you feeling a bit peckish. This is completely normal, a consequence of you shifting your energy system from external to internal sourcing. You're now in the fat-burning zone, where your body is generating its own energy from its stock of pre-digested proteins and fats.

If you're feeling the need for "a little something", the best things to reach for are the various nuts, seeds and fruits from my Top Ten Snacks chart. These nibbles are higher in protein and lower in carbohydrates than your average snack. Nuts in particular are full of protein, fibre and healthy mono-unsaturated and omega-3 fats, while containing very low quantities of carbohydrate. Include mid-morning and mid afternoon snack breaks as part of your Nitro+ daily routine, something to look forward to. This will help to stabilize your energy levels, blood sugars and, by maintaining your positive nitrogen balance, it will also stop you craving things like cream cakes and crisps.

Remember, the important thing is to keep your body's fat burning switch activated and fixed to the ON position.

When should I eat carbohydrates?

Breakfast is the most important meal of the day, and, as we've learned, the best breakfast for fat loss is a small protein feast – 25-30 grams of protein with no carbohydrate. Enjoy a small snack round about elevenses time. Wait until lunchtime before serving up carbohydrates – this should be about half your daily quota of low GL carbs, together with about one third of your daily protein allowance. Lunchtime is the best time to consume half of your low GL carbohydrates, as you'll be burning off more calories for energy in the afternoon. Don't forget to treat yourself to a mid-afternoon snack and make sure that your high protein supper happens before 8 pm.

> *Nitro+ Principle # 11*
> **Consume 35% of your carbo-**
> **hydrates at lunch**

Biological Values

You may have noticed in my Top Ten Protein table a reference to Biological Value. This is to remind us that not all protein foods give the same quality of nutrition. Some are clearly better than others. Proteins with a high bio-logical value are those best suited to maintaining muscle tissue and burning body fat.

Are you ready for a bit more science?

Proteins are composed of 21 biological amino acids. Nine of these are 'essential amino acids', which means that our bodies are incapable of producing them, so we must obtain these from our food intake. The essential amino acids are phenylalanine (25 milligrams per kg of body weight), leucine (39), lysine (30), valine (26), threonine (15), methionine (15), isoleucine (20), histidine (10), and tryptophan (4). When we digest protein, it breaks down into its amino acids, enabling the body to use each for specific purposes. When a protein contains the essential amino acids in a proportion similar to that required by the body, it has a high Biological Value. When one or more of the essential amino acids are missing or present in low numbers, the protein has a low biological value. Unlike carbs or fats that can be stored in the body for future use, unused proteins are excreted. Thus, consuming a lot of low BV protein is not going to be a very efficient way of gaining essential nutrition.

A protein containing all nine essential amino acids is defined as complete; those proteins missing any of these are said to be incomplete.

Vegetables can be complete proteins

Well, fancy that! I'll bet that took you by surprise. Despite what you might have thought, some vegetable proteins are complete, featuring the full spectrum of amino acids.

The chart below indicates the amount of each of the nine essential amino acids in various common vegetables, relative to the body's absolute need.

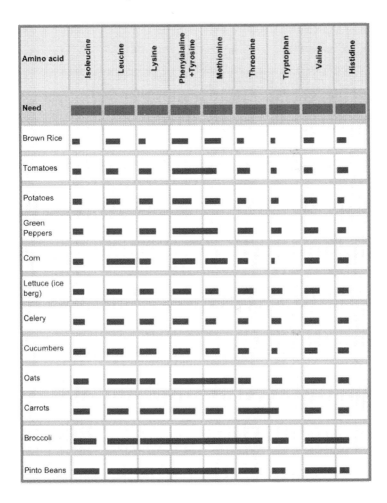

Sources: amino acid need from the World Health Organization, food composition from the USDA nutrient database.

This might contradict some things you've heard down the pub! Vegetables **can** be complete proteins – you just need to select the right ones. Beans, carrots, tomato, celery and even iceberg lettuce are a complete protein – it turns out they are packed with all nine essential amino acids, allowing them to play a key role in maintaining a positive nitrogen balance.

Vegetable protein digestibility

Yes, it's true that experts used to think that vegetable protein is less digestible than protein in beef and fish. I'd like to set the record straight right now. Beef and fish have around 94% digestibility, which is actually less than plant foods such as white flour (96%) and peanut butter (95%). Coming up not far behind – 86-88% – are peas, rice, whole corn, soy flour, oatmeal, and wholewheat flour. Beans, despite their high protein content, are a bit further down on the digestibility scale at 78%. So, it's time to let go of the idea that veg are for wimps. Fact is, vegetables are very good for you, a major help in creating a healthy positive nitrogen balance.

The second measure of protein quality is the protein-digestibility amino acid score (PCDAAS). Quite a mouthful in itself! The PCDAAS method is based on human amino acid requirements, and is recommended by many health officials as the most useful benchmark. A PCDAAS of 1.00 (or 100%) is optimal. Any lower and the protein must be combined with another source containing enough of the missing amino acids to level up the score. Protein sources with a PCDAAS of less than 1.00 typically come from plant sources or fish.

An ideal protein source would have a BV of 70 or higher and a PCDAAS of 1.00, ensuring that your body has the best quality protein and the essential acids it needs to create the positive nitrogen balance that's going to propel you clear into the fat-burning zone. Eggs definitely fall into this category. Here's a handy tip: when scrambling eggs just put in one yolk to 3 egg whites, then mix with either skimmed cows milk or soya milk. The reason? Egg yolks contain a high amount of cholesterol and saturated fat. The same is true of red meat, which is a good reason for limiting this to once per week.

A couple more things: when cooking poultry and meats it's best to steam or oven-cook rather than fry; with vegetables steaming is best.

Fibre: nature's fat torch

Not everything we eat has nutritional value, but that needn't mean it's just a waste of space. Fibre, for example, performs a fantastic job for us. Not only does it regulate insulin metabolism, flattening the insulin peaks and troughs, but it also slows down the digestion of sugars and fats, reducing overall pressure on the system. Increasing your levels of fibre to around 30-50 grams per day can optimize your conversion of food into energy, creating a slow, even uptake, instead of a mad rush to the fat storage parking lot. You'll stay energized, without crashing into that mid-day torpor.

Substantial research has been conducted to evaluate the effect of dietary fibre on body weight, almost all of which show an inverse relationship between dietary fibre intake and change in body weight – the more fibre you eat, the fewer pounds you add on. For example, Tucker and Thomas, in a study involving 252 middle aged women over a 20 month period, observed that participants lost an average of 4.4 pounds. They ascribed this weight loss to an 8 gram increase in dietary fibre per 1000 kcal. This isn't a huge amount of fibre – just 16 grams a day in a 2000 calorie daily diet. Most significant, from our perspective, was that a high percentage of this weight loss was body fat. The researchers noted that the correlation between dietary fibre and weight change was independent of many other potential factors including age, baseline fibre and fat intakes, activity level, and baseline energy intake.

Nitro+ Principle # 12
Consume 30-50 grams of fibre per day

Where can we get this fibre from? No mystery here – all sorts of foods contain an element of fibre.

Just for a change, here comes a Top Sixteen, my choice of high fibre foods. You should aim to consume between 30-50 grams per day as part of your Nitro+ Diet.

It's worth noting how significantly fruit and green vegetables feature in this list.

Top 16 high fibre foods

Food	Fibre per cup (grams)
Split Peas (cooked)	16.3
Lentils (cooked)	15.6
Black Beans (cooked)	15
Lima Beans (cooked)	13.2
Artichoke (cooked) – per vegetable	10.3
Peas (cooked)	8.8
Broccoli (cooked)	5.1
Brussels Sprouts (cooked)	4.1
Raspberries (raw)	8
Blackberries (raw)	7.6
Avocados (raw)	6.7
Pears (raw)	5.5
Bran Flakes (raw)	7
Whole Wheat Pasta	6.3
Pearl Barley	6
Oatmeal	4

- *Make sure you consume protein at every main meal (breakfast, lunch, dinner)*
- *Consume high fibre, low GL foods for lunch and dinner.*

Food integration

You may have come across all sorts of diets referring to food combining, busy drawing up rules on what foods you should or shouldn't eat in combination. To cut the story short, what they agree on is the need to avoid refined carbohydrates, not to mix protein with carbohydrate intake, to consume more alkaline based foods and to eat fruit on its own.

To help us make sense of all this (if you don't mind heading back to science class), let's take a brief look at the science of digestive process.

Digesting protein

· *Eat these first, before your carbohydrates.*

We've already looked at how the body metabolizes carbohydrate into glucose, then into glycogen and fat. Protein digestion happens rather differently. It's a slow, gradual process. When it reaches the stomach, protein is broken down into amino acids by protease enzymes, with the help of strong stomach acid (hydrochloric). The peptide bonds holding the amino acids together are then gradually split apart by the enzyme pepsin, enabling the removal of individual amino acids from the ends of the polypeptide chains. Further along, in the small intestine, more peptidases more or less complete the process of conversion of the protein into amino acids, which can then be transported into the bloodstream.

Personally, I'm not recommending keeping protein and carbohydrate consumption strictly apart. Fact is, you can combine proteins with carbohydrates, although protein is best eaten first, to give the stomach a chance to get busy before carbohydrates or fats start to soak up the acid. Moreover, starting your meal with protein will reduce the blood sugar and insulin spike that typically occurs after eating most refined carbohydrates. In consequence, your blood sugar and insulin levels will stabilise.

Eating protein first may also promote weight loss, as the message "I'm feeling full" reaches the brain faster than it would after commencing with other foods. I'm inviting you to check this out – it works! It's just one of those little changes you can make in your daily routine which are going to make all the difference in the effort to control your weight.

Over 30 days, allow these changes to develop into habits. Stick to the Nitro+ Principles and I guarantee you'll have shaken off those unwanted pounds by the end of this time. You'll be a happier, healthier bunny.

Digesting carbohydrates

When it comes to carbs, digestion is started as soon as it hits your lips. How does the old saying go?. . . a second on the lips and a lifetime on the hips. Now, just think of something tasty: that saliva in your mouth is, technically speaking, the digestive enzyme amylase.

Once swallowed, the food heads down to the stomach, where the stomach acid is waiting to get busy. It's a bit like a breaker's yard, stripping things down to more basic, useable components. You can lend a hand – or, more accurately, your own trusty set of gnashers – by making sure things are properly chewed first.

Take your time eating – this is something we can definitely learn from our continental friends. Over there, mealtimes can be leisurely affairs, a stately progression over one or two hours. It's a big contrast to the fast food culture we've gotten used to, as we ply our hectic lifestyle. Stuff it in your face, wash it down with sugary fizz . . . all over in ten minutes, then back to work! It's really not something to be proud of.

The main business of carbohydrate digestion and absorption takes place in the small intestine, converting the starch into sugars by means of the pancreatic enzyme amylase. For most starches this is a fairly rapid procedure, although some, such as potato, beans, oats and wheat flour, can be more resistant, requiring further attention as they pass into the large intestine, or colon.

That is basically how carbohydrate is digested. I would recommend consuming your carbohydrates AFTER your protein.

> ### Nitro+ Principle # 13
> ## Eat your proteins before your carbohydrates and don't drink fluids with your meal

Snack on fruits and nuts

Fruit, in my opinion, is best eaten on its own. When eaten in combination with other foods it will rot and ferment in your stomach, which can be an uncomfortable experience.

Lower GL fruits are particularly easy to digest. By the time they reach your stomach, digestion is already well under way.

As long as you follow the Nitro+ Diet, with a protein-rich breakfast, you won't be driven to distraction by hunger pangs midway through the mornings and after-noons. Fruit and nuts are going to keep you ticking over nicely.

Animal Protein

Animal protein on its own, which includes not just meat and fish, but also hard cheese and eggs, is also best consumed separately, since these proteins require a lot of stomach acid to digest. If you are going to eat any carbohydrates with animal protein make sure it has a low GL and is not refined or simple sugar.

I'd like to remind you once again not to eat red meat more than once a week, due to the high levels of saturated fats it contains.

New data shows substantial benefits in removing or reducing the consumption of red meat. Not only does red meat increase your risk of colon cancer, it can also shorten your life. That's something to bear in mind next time you're feeling tempted by a burger – or by pork, lamb, and processed meat such as bacon, hot dogs, sausages and salami.

I hate to cast a dampener on your barbie fun, but a recent study involving 84,000 women and 38,000 men found that those who ate the most red meat tended to die younger, particularly from cardiovascular disease and cancer. Specifically, each additional 3 ounce serving of red meat increased risk of death by 13%, while the danger quotient for processed meats rose to a worrying 20%. So how does your mighty whopper burger look now?

Just by substituting red meat with another healthier protein you can reduce your risk . . . by quite a lot. Take a look at these statistics:

Red meat substitute	Reduced risk (%-age)
Fish	7%
Legumes, low fat dairy	10%
Poultry, whole grains	14%
Nuts	19%

www.health.harvard.edu/staying-healthy/cutting-red-meat-for-a-longer-life

Nitro+ Principle # 14
Reduce consumption of red and processed meats

Hydration

Always keep yourself well hydrated throughout the day but avoid drinking your water (or anything else for that matter) while you are eating. Why is this?

It's time to head back to the classroom again – no fidgeting at the back, please!

Although drinking cold water can speed up your metabolism it does so at some cost: bringing the cold water up to body temperature diverts energy that ought to be devoted to the business of digestion. Proteins in particular require a lot of energy to break them down into usable nutrients. Cold water is simply a distraction to the important job that needs doing!

Water can also dilute your nutrients and give you wind, which is not good if you are eating in a fancy restaurant.

Even less recommended, of course, is sluicing down your meal with supersized beakerful after beakerful of sugary pop. Do I really need to mention this again? Sugary beverages as a constant companion to your daily routine really are a no-no. I know the body seems to be saying yes – it's because it just loves a quick and easy carbohydrate fix. That's simply how we have evolved. Our cavemen ancestors, busy chasing down creatures of the wild for their high-grade protein, stashed away whatever carbs they could lay their hands on. Fat was their essential energy resource. But evolution has moved along. Whatever the body seems to be saying, the sensible thing now is simply to say "no, thanks". Sugar is just going to make you fat.

Don't drink liquids with your meals

Good grief! Not even my favourite crispy cabernet sauvignon? Have we given up on civilisation completely?

Well, you can always wait until the kids have gone to bed. Fact is, drinking liquids during your meal dilutes your naturally occurring digestive enzymes and stomach acids, making it harder to break down your food. The saliva produced in the process of chewing should provide quite enough liquid to swallow comfortably. This is why I recommend chewing your food well.

151

It may not be wine, but at least it's wet!

Not to worry, all is not lost. You can have a drink when you are eating! It's not wine or beer, but hey, at least it's wet. You can treat yourself to warm ginger tea or lemon. Ginger is a fantastic tea to drink with or after meals because it naturally moves food from the upper part of the digestive tract into the lower.

You do need to be a little strict here, because it is going to make a lot of difference to how you look in the mirror. And if you keep well hydrated throughout the day you won't be craving sugary drinks at meal times.

Nitro+ Diet tips: a handy summary

- Eat your proteins before your carbohydrates
- Eat your fruits on their own
- Eat healthy protein, preferably on its own or with low GL carbohydrates
- Reduce your consumption of red meat
- Don't drink water or other cold drinks with your food

Nitro+ Principle # 15
Consume NO carbohydrates after 8 pm

I'm going to write this all over again, it's that important.

Consume NO carbohydrates after 8 pm

If you need some help remembering this, here are a few ideas. You could make it into a screen saver. You could paint in on your living room wall (right over your telly). Fix a sign on your fridge door. Just don't forget!

But . . . but . . . what about snacks before bedtime? My hot chocolate to help me snooze? Maybe this sounds really difficult, but, honestly, late night carbohydrate food or drinks are not doing you any favours.

If you are craving sugars or salts late at night it's more than likely because you are dehydrated. It may seem hard – the first few weeks will be the hardest – but, trust me, those hunger pangs will go away.

Why is eating carbs late in the evening so bad? As we've learned, carbohydrates are the body's most readily available source of energy. And there's only so much storage space for the glycogen before it starts getting stashed away as fat.

Do you remember the water analogy I came up with earlier? When the cup (liver) and saucepan (muscles) storage zones are full, water starts to spill over into the bathtub, the infinite fat storage. It's just the way we have evolved; we stash away the energy just in case we ever run out of food.

Eating carbs is also going to set off an insulin spike, as the body reacts to the increased blood sugar levels. This is going to interfere with your natural processes of self repair: human growth hormone (HGH) and insulin growth factor (IGF-1) tend to be produced at night, but insulin in your system will prevent them from setting about their important business.

In the absence of late night carbs, the body goes into something of a closedown metabolic state, running down your liver and muscle glycogen levels over the course of the night. Towards the end of your 7-8 hour sleep the fat burning switch is actually clicked on for a short period, allowing the release of fatty acids to fuel the heart, muscles and liver.

Eating proteins for breakfast is going to keep this fat burning process going, helping you to clear out even more of the visceral fat (the stuff that's packed between your internal organs) that you'd be best off without.

PNB – positive nitrogen balance

It may well be that you think PNB refers to peanut butter, but what I'd like to tell you about is actually quite important. Nitrogen balance is something that body builders and gym obsessives tend to get rather passionate about, and here's the reason why. Muscles can be built up by stressing them with weights, but only when they are in a positive nitrogen balance, which is the consequence of a diet high in quality proteins.

There are three basic states of nitrogen balance:

Positive

This is the optimal state for building up muscle and creating an anabolic environment. It means that nitrogen intake is greater than nitrogen output. When we are in a positive nitrogen balance (PNB) our muscles are much more receptive to nutrients and harder to break down. Okay, maybe bodybuilding isn't really your thing, but hang on in there – things will soon fall into place . . .

Negative

Most overweight people are in Negative Nitrogen Balance (NNB). It's a direct product of their diet: consuming high carbohydrate foods which fire up the insulin roller coaster, not eating enough protein and failing to get their gluconeogenesis metabolism (see Step 2) out of first gear. Another name for the NNB state is catabolic. The catabolic environment is no good at all when it comes to fat burning.

Equilibrium (Balanced)

This occurs when the input and output are the same. Equilibrium Nitrogen Balance is the bare minimum for maximising fat loss.

Muscles that are constantly in a positive or equilibrium state will slow down the breakdown (catabolism) of muscle tissue. This lean muscle tissue needs a steady supply of calories to stay healthy, which is why maintaining Positive Nitrogen Balance will keep your metabolism moving efficiently at the same time as burning off body fat. PNB, in short, is the sure path to keeping your muscles CONSTANTLY in an anabolic state, the ideal fat burning environment, both while you are at rest and when exercising.

Here's how to get into a positive nitrogen balance

The most important thing is to eat more foods high in protein. The more protein, the more nitrogen. When our muscles are in a PNB many great things happen.

Digestion

Often overlooked when assessing protein in the diet is the amount of energy it requires for digestion, compared to fats and carbohydrates. It's really a big difference, as the graph below, comparing the calories needed to digest one gram of each of these foods, makes clear.

My goodness – this really is an eye opener! Digesting protein requires 500% more calories than the equivalent amount of carbohydrates and a massive 1250% more calories than fat.

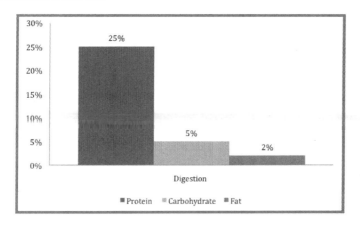

How much calorific energy do organs need?

Take a look at the chart opposite, which tells us how much energy is required per gram for our kidneys, heart, brain, liver, muscles and kidneys.

The heart and kidneys use the most energy per gram, followed by the brain, liver, muscles and heart. By comparison, fat and muscle both require relatively few calories to operate, although as your muscle / fat ratio improves, this will have an effect on your overall calorie expenditure.

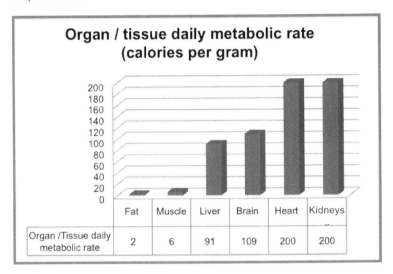

Organ / tissue daily metabolic rate (calories per gram)

	Fat	Muscle	Liver	Brain	Heart	Kidneys
Organ /Tissue daily metabolic rate	2	6	91	109	200	200

Lean muscle tissue

By building lean muscle tissue, you'll be burning far more calories per pound than you would for an equivalent amount of fat. One gram of fat needs 2 calories per day to survive, whereas muscles require around 6 calories. Maybe it doesn't sound like much, but if you gained 7 pounds of muscle (half a stone) and lost 14 pounds of fat (one stone), a net loss of 7 pounds, your extra muscle development would be burning up an additional 70 calories per day. After seven weeks you would have lost a whole pound of fat!

Also, after we've done exercising we'll need to restore our glucose and fat stores, and repair any damaged

The Nitro+ Diet

muscle cells. We'll need more energy, i.e. more calories. Creating these energy gaps is an essential part of the Nitro+ Diet.

Imagine your muscles as a jigsaw. When we exercise and train we remove pieces of this jigsaw. The more gaps we create, the more fat we will use as energy. How? When we exercise, first of all we draw on the glycogen stored in muscle tissue; when this is depleted, we'll need to call upon our deeper energy reserves, which means dipping into our infinite fat storage.

This is why exercise is going to stop you piling on those unwanted pounds.

In summary:

- Consume protein, carbohydrates and fats, according to your Lean Body Mass calculation.
- Create a Positive Nitrogen Balance in your muscles by eating high quality nitrogen foods at all three main meals.
- Avoid the insulin and blood glucose roller coaster by eating low Glycemic Index foods.
- Avoid saturated fats.

Case Study # 4 – Carol

"Carol" was a 37 year old woman, with body fat in the hips, thighs and gluteal areas and a fairly good diet.

The Nitro+ Diet was introduced, kicking off with a 3-4 day detox plan. She commenced weight training, using light weights with a rep range of 15 x 3 sets at least twice per week. Protein was increased and low glycaemic carbohydrates introduced to stabilise blood sugar and suppress the insulin roller coaster.

Before Nitro+ training	
Start weight:	148 lbs
Body fat %-age:	26%
Lean mass:	109 lbs
Fat mass:	39 lbs
Category:	Overweight
After four weeks	
Weight:	141 lbs
Body fat %-age:	22%
Lean mass:	110 lbs
Fat mass:	31 lbs
Category:	Normal

The total weight lost amounted to 7 lbs (half a stone) with body fat reduced by 4% and lean body mass increased by one pound. Carol was delighted with the results and was able to drop a dress size over the course of the 4 week programme!

Step 4 – Ignite

Fat burning countdown is go!

Things are really hotting up here. I hope you can feel the palpable sense of excitement as we prepare to fire up the fat burners, ready for blast off.

We've succeeded in defining the perfect fat burning environment. Now it's time to ignite your muscles and switch the turbo chargers on. Step 4 is going to blast the doors to your fat storage bay wide open, so you get the maximum burn-off.

It's all about exercise. I love exercise, it's great. In fact, I'd say regular exercise is the best feeling in the world. It gets to be addictive, once you see how your body starts to change shape and your overall energy level builds and builds.

I love running, especially in forests. If running doesn't seem possible for you, try walking. Load up your mp3 player with some motivating music and head on outdoors. Exercise will energise you, increase your vitality and provide you with a sense of direction. Remember where you're heading for – rapid, lasting fat loss.

In this chapter we're going to explore a range of things – dietary supplements, lifestyle tips, and exercise techniques – which will help set you up for all systems go.

Chromium

This is the stuff that they used to decorate flash cars with back in the 1950s, but don't worry, we're not going to be eating cars. It happens to be a chemical element, a metal with the symbol Cr, and it does, in very small quantities, play an important role in our metabolism.

We need chromium to regulate the action of insulin, making sure that it's performing its job effectively. This means that it's a significant player in building muscle and controlling body fat, because insulin has such a big influence on the uptake of glucose and amino acids. It helps in controlling hunger, reducing sugar cravings and suppressing appetite. Your muscles will be all the happier for it, which in turn will have a long-term positive effect on your metabolism.

Sad to say, chromium deficiency is widespread, but fortunately it is available as a dietary supplement. I recommend taking 200 mcg of chromium supplement daily – this should really fire you up. Your insulin levels will be stabilised, slowing down the insulin roller coaster. You will feel more energised, with fewer periods of tiredness. Thanks to its beneficial effects on insulin performance, digestion of protein will be improved, allowing more amino acids to be taken up by muscle tissue, and therefore facilitating muscle build-up. Chromium also has anabolic effects and can help keep your muscles in a positive nitrogen balance.

The body is such a complex interactive process! Make sure everything it needs is present, and lift-off is going to become so much easier.

How much difference could a little chromium make? A study was carried out at the Bemidgi State University over a period of 6 weeks, comparing two groups, one of which were given a daily dose of 200 mcg chromium picolinate, a type of chromium supplement, the other a placebo. Both groups participated in a resistance training routine. The group that was not taking chromium made negligible gains, whereas the chromium group gained an average of 3.5 pounds of lean, fat burning muscle. A further, larger study followed, to see if these results could be repeated. Over six weeks two groups of football players followed a similar procedure, and the results served to confirm the earlier experiment. The chromium group gained 5.7 pounds of lean body mass compared to 4 pounds for the control group. That's an amazing 40% more lean body mass. Even more impressively, the chromium group lost 3.6% of body fat compared to a mere 1% loss in the control group.

I rest my case!

Zinc

Here's another metal we've reason to be thankful for. Did you ever imagine your body could contain so many different metals? Luckily, these are very tiny quantities, mere traces, certainly not enough to cause you any anxiety as you progress through the airport metal detector.

The importance of zinc in our diet is no big secret. Taken as a supplement it can have very beneficial effects, optimising insulin metabolism and improving insulin sensitivity, thus improving the uptake of sugar into your cells. It bolsters and strengthens our immune system and plays an important role in healing wounds, in stimulating cell growth and during periods of heightened transformation, such as pregnancy and infancy. It's also effective in reducing the risk of catching a cold, and can ease the symptoms when you do.

Some supplements combine zinc with magnesium and vitamin D, a winning combination.

A study published in the 2013 edition of Biological Trace Element Research reported that people who were obese had lower levels of zinc in their bodies. In the same year, another study discussed in the Advanced Pharmaceutical Bulletin found that obese people who had a daily zinc supplement of 30 mg per day experienced improved body mass indices and also lost weight.

You don't have to just rely on supplements: significant levels of zinc are naturally present in high protein foods such as beef, pork and lamb.

Symptoms of zinc deficiency include:

- Poor appetite
- Frequent colds
- Loss of hair
- Cold sores
- Wounds take a long time to heal

Essential Fatty Acids

Omega 3 fatty acids – EFAs – are found in fish oils, and are also available in handy supplement form. They are indeed essential, particularly when you're on a low carb diet such as Nitro+. They'll help to give you energy and to keep your metabolism running optimally – the last thing you want when you're dieting is a slow metabolism! EFAs increase muscle glutamine levels, which can promote protein synthesis. They can also influence growth hormone levels, which in turn can increase muscle nitrogen balance and decrease body fat. Supplementation with EFAs has been proven to significantly decrease chronic rheumatoid arthritis, chronic fatigue symptoms and hypertension.

5-HTP

This supplement is optional, but if you're someone with a sweet tooth then you might find it helpful in reducing those cravings for a certain sugary something.

Also known as oxitriptan, 5-HTP is a naturally occurring amino acid. There's not a lot of research been done on its effects, but I have turned up an Italian study in which a group of overweight or obese adults were placed on a 1,200 calorie diet over a period of 12 weeks. Half the participants were given a dose of 300 milligrams (mg) 30 minutes before each meal, while half were (unknowingly) given a placebo. The results showed that the 5-HTP group lost about 7.2 lbs over the course of the experiment, compared to an average loss of 4 lbs amongst those who took the placebo.

It does seem to be safe and free from unwanted side-effects, although you should avoid it if you are taking anti-depressants, as it interferes with the action of serotonin.

Recommended daily supplement intake

Chromium Picolinate*	200 mcg (with breakfast)
Zinc Picolinate*	30 mg (with breakfast)
EFAs*	1.5 g - 2 g (in the morning)
5-HTP (optional)*	300 mg before meals

---

*   *For in depth information on contraindications, side effects and interactions for any of these supplements please check the Supplement Contraindications section at the back of this book. If in doubt please consult your doctor or physician.*

Nitro+ Principle # 16
Maintain daily recommended intake of chromium, zinc, and fish oil

---

L-carnitine

Ring ring goes the bell . . . yes, it's back to the classroom again! We're going to look at what happens after you've created the perfect fat burning environment, and find out how you can ratchet up the effect by a few more gears.

Pull open your mental microscope, and take a look at what's happening inside your muscle cells. There are tiny structures known as mitochondria which busy themselves burning up fats. In effect they are the cells' internal power-house. In order for this process to occur, the adipose cells containing the fats need to be accompanied by the amino acid L-carnitine, otherwise they are unable to cross into the mitochondrial matrix. Basically, the higher the levels of L-carnitine, the higher the amount of body fat which can be accessed for fuel.

L-carnitine is an amino acid that can be easily sourced from any health store. Remember that massive, unlimited storage where your surplus fat gets locked away? Now imagine it as a room full of doors ready to be opened. L-carnitine will provide the key.

A 2013 clinical study has attracted a great deal of attention. It showed that dietary supplementation of 500 mg L-carnitine per day, in combination with exercise training, was enough to ensure significant weight loss in over-weight individuals. Study participants were able to lose an average of 400 g of body fat within four weeks, without otherwise changing their diets or level of exercise. Waist circumference measurements showed an average decrease of 1.3 cm (just over half an inch). I hope you're impressed – nearly half a kilo of dangerous visceral fat gone in one month, simply by taking a half a gram of L-carnitine. And your pants are going to stop feeling quite so tight!

Sounds good to me.

In another piece of research, two scientists from Switzerland and the USA demonstrate that the adminis-tration of L-carnitine can boost mobilization of fatty acids from the adipocytes (fat cells) and also increase oxidation of fatty acids in these cells.

Moreover, sufficient data has been obtained from seven animal models which all clearly indicate that L-carnitine supplementation during a calorie-reduced diet can lead not only to a significant decrease in the body fat compared to a placebo, but also to a simultaneous increase in fat-free muscle mass.

Impressed? Now check this out!

Here's another impressive piece of research, this time by Gilbert Kaats of Health and Medical Services of San Antonio, Texas. In this trial, groups of five overweight men and women were first given low fat diets of 1250 calories for women and 1650 for men over a period of eight weeks. This reduced calorie diet resulted in very little weight loss. Subsequently, over a further eight weeks, their diets were augmented by the following supplements:

- Chromium Picolinate   400 mcg
- L-carnitine   200 mcg
- Fibre   20 grams

At the end of this second period, subjects showed an average weight loss of 15.1 lbs, of which fat loss amounted to 11.8 lbs. How amazing is that – over a whole stone, just gone! Now, I am not guaranteeing that you're going to drop a whole stone by following this particular procedure, but it certainly does demonstrate the importance of chromium, L-carnitine and fibre in your diet.

Nitro+ Principle # 17
Consume 500 mg-1000 mg L-carnitine daily

Drink Green Tea

Cranking up your metabolism isn't all about exploring the further frontiers of science. What's the most everyday means of perking yourself up? That's right – a lovely cup of steaming rosie lee. But there's a twist (maybe of lemon?). Green tea is the stuff to go for, if you want to make the most of this mighty beverage.

There are all sorts of health benefits to drinking green tea, including lowering blood pressure and keeping blood sugar levels stable, but what we're chiefly interested in here is the ability of green tea to inhibit fat absorption.

A study published in the American Journal of Clinical Nutrition reported that consuming an extract of green tea can increase your metabolic rate by an amazing 4% over a 24 hour period. Drinking just three to five cups a day can burn off as much as 70 calories per day. This may not sound much, but over a year this could add up to seven pounds – half a stone! – an impressive vanishing act, fuelled simply by a few cups daily of the cup that cheers.

And if drinking tea really isn't your bag, you could always try a green tea supplement.

http://www.bodybuilding.com/fun/9-tips-to-increase-metabo-lism.htm

Recommended daily dosages	
L-Carnitine *	500 g -1000 g daily
Green Tea*	2-3 cups per day

* For in depth information on contraindications, side effects and interactions for any of these supplements please check the Supplement Contraindications section at the back of this book. If in doubt please consult your doctor or physician.

Nitro+ Principle # 18
Drink 2-3 cups of green tea daily (or equivalent supplement) to boost your metabolism.

Crank up your metabolism with caffeine

Caffeine cranks up the metabolism and can therefore help burn off more body fat – so this is good news for all those who enjoy the caffeine kick contained in a nice cup of coffee. You're certainly not in a minority – caffeine happens to be the most commonly used psychoactive substance in the world. It's come a long way since its origins in the medieval Ethiopian kingdom of Kaffa.

These days we're spoiled for choice, with so many shops on the high street offering a bewildering variety of speciality brews from all round the world. The coffee bar has taken the place of the pub as the preferred place to socialise, to host business meetings and to engage in networking. Starbucks alone operates more than 21,000 outlets around the world.

Never mind trying to make your mind up between lattes, cappucinos, frappucinos, all that business with frothed-up milk; what's really going to help your weight loss regime is straightforward black coffee. It's truly a metabolic powerhouse, combining a range of biologically active substances, including:

- **Caffeine.** As is well known, this acts as a stimulant to the central nervous system. It can also increase the levels of the hormone epinephrine (better known as adrenaline). When epinephrine travels in the blood-stream it facilitates the breakdown of fat cells into free fatty acids, enabling stored fat to be mobilised as energy.
- **Theobromine and theophylline**. These are related to caffeine and can have a stimulant effect.
- **Chlorogenic acid.** There are reports that this acid, a biologically active compound, can slow down the absorption of carbohydrates.

All in all, this amazing substance has been shown to increase the metabolic rate by between 3 and 11%, mostly a result of burning fat for energy, although this effect is less pronounced in those who are obese. Another great benefit of caffeine is that it can suppress your appetite and help you eat less.

It is worth bearing in mind that the body quite rapidly gains a tolerance for caffeine, so that it becomes less effective over a longer term.

I would certainly recommend drinking one or two cups of black coffee a day, to crank up the metabolism and facilitate fat loss. You can lay off those fancy cappuccinos, lattes and mochas, though. These dairy rich drinks are far too loaded down with calories! Go for the espresso and you won't be disappointed; if you must add something to whiten it up, try soy milk – my guess is you won't even notice the difference.

> ## *Nitro+ Principle # 19*
> # Crank up your metabolism with caffeine

Conjugated Linoleic Acid

Yes I know, this is a bit of a mouthful, so to make things easy we can just talk about CLA and we'll know what we're about.

This really is a fantastic supplement, which melts away the body fat despite being itself a fat. CLA is closely related to the omega-6 fatty acids and can help reduce bad cholesterol, strengthen the immune system and boost the metabolism. It can also improve concentration and sleep. It occurs naturally in dairy and meat products.

From our point of view, the great thing about CLA is that it can burn fat and build muscle. Don't forget, we want to hang on to our muscles, as these are our body's engines and fat burners. Once you have lost fat CLA will help maintain your weight and keep the fat at bay. Taken together with the low glycaemic foods mentioned in Step 3, CLA has a big part to play in igniting your fat burning capabilities.

I recently came across a study entitled "Conjugated linoleic acid reduces body fat mass in overweight and obese humans". This demonstrated that those participants taking the supplement experienced a significant reduction in body fat mass, although doses larger than 3.4 g per day led to no additional effect on body fat.

This study clearly shows the benefits of taking CLA, describing its effects on lipolysis in adipose cells (the breakdown of fat in fat cells to free fatty acids), and its promotion of increased fatty acid oxidation from stored fat in both adipocytes and skeletal muscle. Thrice daily (before breakfast, lunch and dinner) consumption of CLA enabled overweight and obese participants to increase lean body mass slightly, decrease body fat mass significantly and improve muscular strength.

Nitro+ Principle # 20
Consume CLA to burn fat and to stop it coming back

We're well on our way to creating the perfect fat burning environment. Here are some more recommended daily intakes*.

Recommended daily intake	
CLA	One tablet (1 g), three times daily, before meals
Black coffee	1 - 2 cups per day

*   *For in depth information on contraindications, side effects and interactions for any of these supplements please check the Supplement Contraindications section at the back of this book. If in doubt please consult your doctor or physician.*

Fire up your engine with the Kinetic Workout Plan

Before we launch into the sweaty business of stretches and lunges, let's do a bit of a recap.

Your body's engine runs on glucose, not calories. Glucose comes from the food you eat, but if you reduce the levels of easily accessible glucose as a result of following the Nitro+ Diet, the energy is going to have to come from the reserves of stored fat. You'll be burning it off, to produce a trimmer, slimmer you.

The Kinetic workout plan is designed to raise your fat burning rate by switching on the muscles, your fat burning engines. Active, toned muscle will call up the necessary nutrients to allow movement or exercise and burn body fat as fuel. Using the Bellmate Kinetic for just 25 minutes per day, three days per week, whilst following the Nitro+ Diet will burn off body fat at an incredible rate and transform your physique – in just one month.

Amongst the benefits of this Nitro+ Diet are:

- Stronger bones
- Reduced blood pressure
- Lower HDL (bad cholesterol)
- Higher LDL (good cholesterol)
- Improved heart health
- Reduced risk of diabetes and arthritis
- Improved muscle tone
- Improved posture
- Improved joint health

- Stronger core muscles
- Improved cardiovascular system

It's time to turn on your ignition!

People are eating more than ever, not exercising enough and getting fatter. By 2050 half of the developed world will be overweight or obese. Despite there being more gyms than ever we aren't getting nearly enough exercise. What's going on here?

I think that there has been a bit of a stigma attached to weight training. Perhaps the whole Mr Universe image of bodybuilding isn't as sexy as it once might have been. Women in particular tend to avoid weights, as they don't want to get muscular or bulk up. But let's not forget what we're about. Muscles are crucial to our Kinetic revolution – the means to keep us lean

It's not as easy as you might think to build muscles. The weights need to be heavy, with a rep range of 6-10, testosterone plays a large part and you will need large amounts of protein. When we don't use our muscles, we lose them – use it or lose it, as the old saying goes. This is clear enough when we look at many elderly folk: their muscles have wasted away, their posture is poor, with forward head flexion, and they find it hard to get around. But even at this stage of life, all is not lost. Studies have been carried out on weight training for the elderly, with amazing results. It's clear that strength and weight training does make you younger. Yep, that's right, younger! And that's not all – weight training can improve:

- Strength and muscle mass
- Blood lipids
- Body composition
- Bone density
- Aerobic capacity
- Blood pressure
- Cardiorespiratory fitness

Blood glucose & cardiovascular disease

Remember how the body stores glucose and how we store fat? When you can control your glucose levels you can lower your risk of cardiovascular disease by as much as 42%. Weight training is going to play a major role in this process.

A typical weight-training workout might use around 35-60 grams of carbohydrates and eat into the readily available glycogen storage. When you start to drain this system, it makes room for more glycogen to be stored: this is known as super compensation. Simply by following the Nitro+ Diet together with the Kinetic Fit system for a total of just 40-45 minutes per week (in three 12-15 minute workouts), you will be able to create this super compensation environment. You'll be activating stored reserves of body fat to use as energy at the same time as developing a handy bit of available storage in your muscles and liver. Instead of being bundled off into storage, carbohydrates will be used up as fuel for your muscles. Your body composition will change – and quickly.

Osteoporosis

As we get older, our bones become weaker. The average 30-35 year old is likely to experience a 25% decline in their muscles by the age of 70-75 and a 50% decline by the age of 90. Weight training is a good way to slow down this process and stay functional for longer; it can reduce the onset of bone loss and even, according to some studies, actually build bone. Weight training is one of the best things you can do to slow down the onset of osteoporosis. Go for it!

Forbes Magazine February 10, 2013
Mercola

Exercise and fitness

First an important word or two from our reality check inspector. High intensity exercise is not suitable for everyone. If in any doubt that you are fit enough, please consult your doctor before commencing the Nitro+ Diet or exercise programme.

If all seems well, I invite you to celebrate your commitment to a new healthier lifestyle by throwing out your comfortable loafers and investing in a pair of decent trainers. Exercise is going to make you feel so much better. It's going to fill you with energy. Give it a go –you can thank me later!

Blimey! So what happens now?

I'm going to describe two different types of workout, the anabolic and the catabolic. Each has a different effect on your body but both will ultimately lead to fat loss.

If I can jog your memory: in terms of biochemistry,

anabolic is about creating complex molecules from simpler ones. So the anabolic workouts are designed to build up muscle mass, at the same time as shedding fat. Catabolic, in contrast, involves breaking down complexity into simpler structures; the consequent release of heat can itself be the motor of anabolic process. Catabolic exercise is going to reduce your overall body mass. In combination, you can achieve fast and long-lasting weight loss. I'll be describing a selection of exercises in a short while.

Weight training: the best anabolic workout

Why do most overweight people, when they get to the gym, make a beeline for the cardio room? I reckon it's because they believe running, cycling, cross training or rowing will burn off the body fat – but they're making a big mistake. It's not that some fat doesn't burn off; it does, though not by much. The fact is, to get into an anabolic state you need to focus on strength training, in order to increase muscle mass.

Strength training will stimulate testosterone (in men) and growth hormone and will induce both muscle soreness and growth – anabolism, in short. It's a process of stress and release: with the help of weights and machines, the muscles are overloaded and resistance developed; afterwards, in the period of rest or sleep following your workout, you'll experience the release of hormones, as well as the high that comes from an elevated heightened metabolic state. Some experts reckon that your metabolism remains raised for as much as 39 hours following weight training.

Cardio is catabolic

Cardio is another way of talking about aerobics. Many catabolic exercises involve cardiovascular techniques, usually lasting at least 20 to 45 minutes at low intensity. Examples are cycling, running, swimming and playing sports.

The catabolic process involves a different set of hormones to anabolic – in this case cortisol, norepinephrine and adrenalin. These get busy burning fat and calories, with the end result being a loss of total body mass.

These cardio exercises provide an excellent way to give the cardiovascular system a sustained workout (typically 15-20 minutes for an aerobic session), using oxygen as a fuel source. Cardio exercises will also raise your metabolism.

HIIT training

HIIT is short for high intensity interval training. You might think it's the new kid on the exercise block, but actually it's been around for a while, under a variety of different names.

High intensity interval training involves going flat out for 30 seconds and then resting for 1-2 minutes. By flat out, I mean more than 85% of your maximum heart rate. I find it easiest to do HIIT training on an exercise bike. Set the bike at a mid level and do one minute easy and then go full power for 30 seconds; take the next two minutes at a slow pace, then hit the throttle again. Repeat the process four or five times – as your fitness improves, you can experiment with reducing your rest time and increasing the full-on section.

HIIT training is fantastic for creating an anabolic environment and burning body fat. However, high intensity intervals can be tough on the body and are not recommended for everyone. Consult your doctor and ask a gym instructor for a health check (blood pressure etc). If there's a green flag, on your bike and off you go! It'll all be over in 10-12 minutes.

http://www.bodybuilding.com/fun/9-tips-to-increase-metabolism.htm

Combination of weight training and cardio is best

My recommendation is to combine anabolic with catabolic workouts to shred body fat and stay fit.

Performing both anabolic and catabolic exercises provides you with variety in your workout routine. Not only will you avoid getting bored, but you'll be continuously shocking your metabolism into shedding fat and burning calories. You can add intensity to your workouts by using each approach either alternately or simultaneously.

> *Nitro+ Principle # 21*
>
> **Introduce resistance training 3 times per week, with small cardio intervals**

Top Fat Burning Exercises

Introducing the Bellmate Kinetic

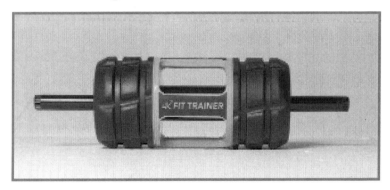

Excuse me while I get excited. Just take a look at this! The Bellmate Kinetic is an innovative piece of kit that's just great for developing overall body fitness and enabling fat loss. It's an all-in-one technological marvel, packed with special features.

Here's some of the things it can do: the tyre tread outer casing is great for trigger point release, allowing you to unpack your muscles; pull out the handles and you have an abdominal roller and barbell; pop the handles back in and you've got a dumbbell and kettle bell. It's practically a whole gym, in one stylish, highly portable box. Plus, it comes fully equipped with optional adjustable weights, a bag, a mat and gloves! Just log onto our website and click on the shop icon.

The Kinetic is available in a range of attractive colours. It's weight adjustable from 3 to 5 Kg and measures just over 30 cm across – that's the same length as a foot ruler.

In short, it's eminently portable – it might even fit in your handbag!

Spend just 75 minutes per week – three 25 minute sessions – doing these exercises and you'll succeed in igniting your muscles, turning them into turbo-charged fat burning engines, capable of transforming your fat storage into energy.

Do I hear you saying, you just don't have the time? C'mon, 25 minutes every other day, let's get serious! Get up a little earlier, make sure you don't hit the snooze button on your alarm clock – if you snooze you lose. This is too good to miss!

For warm up stretches, cool downs and over 200 video exercises (including those described below) go to our website and claim your FREE ONE MONTH ACCESS to the complete Kinetic Fit System.

Exercise # 1
Clean and Press

This is my favourite exercise, a compound movement utilising a combination of muscles. It will build strength, head to toe stability and develop explosive power. This exercise is ideal for many sports due to its ballistic move-ment and dynamic nature. It's also great for overall fitness, an effective training for the cardiovascular system.

1. Standing with your shins almost touching the Kinetic (ensure handles are in the out position) or barbell, with feet shoulder width apart, use an overhand grip to grasp the kinetic handles or barbell.

2. Pull your tummy in and activate your core muscles. If using the Kinetic, keep the foam pressed against your body and drive through your heels while pushing the hips forward.

3. Pull the Kinetic or barbell past your hips, rising up on your tiptoes and shrugging your shoulders, leading with the elbows.

4. When the Kinetic or barbell is at shoulder height, using momentum rotate the elbows under the bar.

5. The Kinetic/barbell is now at shoulder height under full control. Extend it directly above your head by locking out your arms.

6. Reverse the exercise back to the beginning.

Carry out 3 sets of 12-15 repetitions, allowing for a 30 second rest between sets.

Exercise # 2
Bent Over Row & Deadlift – 'Dead Row'

This is another great compound exercise that builds strength and power, targeting legs, back, core, biceps and shoulders. It's great for improving lower and upper back strength, developing cardiovascular fitness and muscular endurance. I have cleverly named this exercise the Dead Row.

• Position the Kinetic or barbell in front of you on the floor. Take an overhand grip on the handles and stand up tall, contracting your lower back, hamstrings (backs of legs) and pulling your tummy in. This is the deadlift part of the exercise.

- Then hinge at the waist, bending forward, and stick your bottom out as if you're going to sit down on a chair. Allow the arms to hang straight in front of you. Squeeze your shoulder blades together and pull the Kinetic / barbell towards your chest. Hold it on your chest for one second and then lower back down to straight arm position, then stand up straight again. This is one full repetition.

Carry out 3 sets of 12-15 repetitions, allowing for a 30 second rest between sets.

Exercise # 3
Upright Row and Squat

This is a great compound exercise to develop and condition the upper and lower back, biceps (fronts of the arms), shoulders, core and legs.

- Position the Kinetic or barbell in front of you on the floor. Take an overhand grip on the handles or the inside handles on the Kinetic and stand up tall, contracting your lower back, hamstrings (backs of legs) and pulling your tummy in. This is your starting position. As you squat down, simultaneously start the upright row. At the bottom of the squat the Kinetic / barbell will be at chin height, with your elbows facing outwards and your shoulder blades squeezed together. Hold for one second and then return to the beginning.

Carry out 3 sets of 12-15 repetitions, allowing for a 30 second rest between sets.

Exercise # 4
Press Up

This exercise is particularly good on the Kinetic, developing and strengthening the abdominals, core shoulders, arms and back.

- For this exercise it's best to have a mat positioned under your knees. Get on all fours, grab hold of the Kinetic handles and glide the roller out to the front. Be careful not to extend too far forward, otherwise you could injure yourself. When it has rolled out to a comfortable position, complete a press up with elbows pointing outwards. After you have completed the press up, pull the Kinetic back to the starting position.

Carry out 3 sets of 12-15 repetitions, allowing for a 30 second rest between sets.

Exercise # 5
Shoulder Press and Squat

This is another one of my favourite compound exercises. It's very effective at developing and strengthening the whole body, especially the legs, core back, shoulders and arms. This exercise will also develop speed and improve cardiovascular fitness.

- Position the Kinetic or barbell in front of you on the floor. Take an overhand grip on the handles or the inside handles on the Kinetic and stand up tall, contracting your lower back, hamstrings (backs of legs) and pulling your tummy in, then lift the Kinetic / barbell to shoulder height. Engaging the core and with chest out, squat down to around 90° at the knee. Stand up explosively and press the kinetic over your head. Hold the Kinetic steady when arms are locked out, then return back to the starting position.

Carry out 3 sets of 12-15 repetitions, allowing for a 30 second rest between sets.

Exercise # 6
Kinetic Swings

This is one of the best and most popular exercises, a great way to improve your fitness, crank up your metabolism and, in consequence, burn up body fat.

It does great things for the posterior chain – that is, the muscles at the back of the body: your hamstrings (backs of legs), gluteus (bottom) and lower back. If you spend a large part of the day sitting at a desk, then this exercise will be ideal for you. When you are sitting at your desk the muscles of the butt and abdominals become weak while the lower back and hamstrings (backs of legs) start to tighten up and grow shorter. The Kinetic swings will help strengthen and lengthen these muscles.

The upper body is also worked hard, especially the back and shoulders.

There are two types of swing. The American swing takes the Kinetic / kettle bell all the way to above your head, whereas the Russian swing stops at the eye line.

Here I'll be describing the Russian swing, which can be developed into the American swing when you are ready.

If you're intending to lift the Kinetic above your head, make sure there's enough room – I've hit false ceilings many times doing this exercise!

- Bend at the hips and pick up the Kinetic using the central handles. The outside handles can be locked away. Slowly rock the Kinetic between your legs, then, while squeezing your butt muscles (gluteus), thrust your hips forward with speed and swing the Kinetic to eye level, then return the Kinetic back to the starting position and repeat. Ensure that your back is kept straight and that you generate the power from your hips.

Carry out 3 sets of 12-15 repetitions, allowing for a 30 second rest between sets.

Exercise # 7
Kinetic Crunch

This is an exciting new exercise that can only be carried out with the Kinetic. It will work the abdominals harder than ever as well as engaging the core throughout the whole of the exercise.

- Ensure the Kinetic outer handles are pulled out. Lying down on a mat, bend your knees so that the soles of your feet are on the floor. Place the Kinetic on your pelvis, then, keeping your head in one position, lift your shoulders towards the ceiling. Keeping your lower back on the mat, roll the Kinetic to the knee while maintaining pressure on the legs at all times. Exhale at the top of the exercise and slowly roll the Kinetic back down the legs, then repeat. To target the obliques (the muscles to the side of the abdominal wall), take a wider foot stance and roll the Kinetic up one leg at a time – i.e. 10 on the right leg and then 10 on the left leg.

Carry out 3 sets of 12-15 repetitions, allowing for a 30 second rest between sets.

Exercise # 8
Kinetic Lunge Curls

This exercise will tone the butt and legs, activate the core, tone the fronts of the arms (biceps) and improve your balance. Kinetic lunge curls can also improve dynamic flexibility in the hips, knees and ankle joints.

• Pull the handles out of the Kinetic and take an underhand grip (palms facing up). Stand up, holding the Kinetic at hip height. Take a big step out into a lunge while simultaneously curling the Kinetic to shoulder height. Driving off your front big toe, step back to the standing position, at the same time lowering the Kinetic curl. Repeat on the other leg and alternate for 20 repetitions (10 on each leg).

Carry out 3 sets of 12-15 repetitions allowing for a 30 second rest between sets.

Exercise # 9
Kinetic Plank

This popular and effective exercise goes by several different names, including front hold and abdominal bridge, but plank is the most common name. It is a fantastic isometric (held in one position) core strength exercise, which has become a key feature of yoga and pilates classes all round the world. The muscles worked are the back, abdominals, upper back, chest, legs and butt.

• Push the Kinetic handles in. On a mat, get into a press up position and rest your forearms on the Kinetic. Lift your hips off the floor and maintain this position: your body should be straight from your shoulders to your ankles. Activate your core by pulling in your tummy. Hold this position for 30 seconds (increase this time when you improve) and then take a one minute rest. Complete a total of 3 sets for a full body workout.

Carry out 3 sets of 12-15 repetitions allowing for a 30 second rest between sets.

Exercise # 10
Kinetic Wall Squats

This is another fantastic exercise that tones and strengthens the lower back and legs.

- Pull the handles out of the Kinetic and place next to a wall. Stand up straight, with your back against the wall, and position the Kinetic roller behind you at the middle of your back. Bend your knees and roll the Kinetic down the wall for a count of three, until your thighs are parallel to the floor, then hold this position for two seconds. Push through your heels back to the starting position.

Carry out 3 sets of 12-15 repetitions, allowing for a 30 second rest between sets.

189

Your Nitro+ Kinetic Exercise Programme

Three short sessions per week, about 45 minutes in total

- **Day 1**

   3 sets of 15 reps / 30 seconds rest time

   Clean and press

   Bent over row and deadlift

   Upright row and squat

   Kinetic crunches

- **Day 2**

   3 sets of 15 reps / 30 seconds rest time

   Abdominal roller and press up

   Shoulder press and squat

   Kinetic swings

   Kinetic crunches

- **Day 3**

   3 sets of 15 reps / 30 seconds rest time

   Kinetic lunge curls

   Kinetic plank

   Kinetic wall squats

   Kinetic crunches

Complete this workout for just four weeks and you will really notice the difference. You'll look good, and you'll feel great. You'll be able to drop a dress size, or a shirt size, and pull in your belt an extra notch or two. You'll be proud of the photos from the wedding or birthday party – proof for all time of the hard work you've been putting in.

These exercises really are amazing and effective. They will tone and strengthen your muscles, your core, and shape up your butt and legs. In combination with the Nitro+ Diet you'll be igniting your muscles so you can burn off pounds and pounds of unwanted body fat at an amazing rate. So stick with it – there will be big changes, I can guarantee it.

> ### *Nitro+ Principle # 22*
> ### Train three times per week with the Kinetic to ignite your muscles

Trigger Point Release with the Kinetic

The Kinetic is not just a dumbbell, barbell, kettle bell, and abdominal roller; it's also a trigger point release device, great for easing muscular tension. The foam roller has been proven to:

- Improve the range of hamstring motion, from just 10 seconds of usage
- Reduce arterial stiffness and improve flexibility
- Improve balance in older women who used foam rollers in just 5 weeks

Ten sites for trigger point release

For these exercises you can have the Kinetic handles either in or out.

1. IT band (hip to knee)

You hear a lot of people in the gym talking about the IT band, often in connection to hip and knee pain: it gets to carry a lot of blame. It refers to the illotibial band, a ligament running from your hip to the outside of your knee, which can become tight or inflamed. To ease this out, position the Kinetic below your hip, keeping one leg on the floor to stabilize yourself. Gradually work the roller down from the hip to the knee; if you find a tender spot, push down and hold or roll quickly back and forth over the tender spot. This will really help loosen up your ligament.

2. TFL or hip flexor (top and front of thigh)

Spread your legs outwards. Start the Kinetic at your hip and work down to the knee. If you hit a tender area, roll the kinetic over this area several times. This will help release the hip flexors.

3. Quadriceps (thigh)

Position yourself in the press up position, keeping your hands on the floor and core tight. Start with the Kinetic at your hip and roll it down to the knee. This will give the thigh a stretch from the front. You can also do this one when seated – simply pull out the Kinetic handles and roll over the thigh.

4. Hamstrings and gluteus (backs of legs and butt)

With the Kinetic roller on the floor, position your butt

(gluteus) on top and roll your hips and hamstrings over it. This will help release the butt and hamstrings.

5. Calf

The calves, located at the back of the lower leg, can get tight. To ease them out, sit yourself on the ground and position the Kinetic roller underneath the lower leg, then roll backwards and forwards while keeping the legs as straight as possible.

6. Ankle

Ankles do get tight as well. Roll the Kinetic roller on the sides of the ankle or from the anklebone up to mid calf.

7. Latissimus (back muscles)

Everyone knows about achy back muscles. To release these muscles roll the Kinetic roller from the armpit and down your side to the rib cage.

8. Lower back and hip

This provides a nice massage, but do proceed with caution, as these muscles can be tender. Position the Kinetic roller on the floor, then, keeping your shoulders on the floor, roll your hips back and forth over the roller.

9. Upper back

This one is very similar to the previous action. Start with hips on the ground and roll back and forth over the middle of your back.

10.Gluteal

The gluteal muscles are a group of three which make up your buttocks. Position the Kinetic roller on the floor and sit on the roller with both knees bent. Slowly rock back and forth over the roller to help release the butt (gluteus).

Summary

- Exercise regularly: resistance training at least 3 times per week
- Take l -carnitine supplement daily
- Take CLA supplement 3 times per day
- Consume 2-3 cups of green tea per day or take a supplement
- Drink 2-3 cups of black coffee per day
- Take chromium, zinc and EFA on a daily basis

Case Study # 5 – Pamela

Pamela, a 56 year old woman, had problems with body fat in the normal areas but her real difficulties concerned muscle wastage (negative nitrogen balance) and a poor diet.

The Nitro+ Diet was introduced, kicking off with a 3 day detox programme. Weight training commenced, using light weights with a rep range of 15 x 3 sets, at least once per week. The main aim was to switch the muscles back into positive nitrogen balance to allow body fat to be utilised for energy and for general health and mobility.

Before Nitro+ training	
Weight:	125 lbs
Body fat %-age:	28%
Lean mass:	90 lbs
Fat mass:	35 lbs
Category:	Overweight
After eight weeks	
Weight :	117 lbs
Body fat %-age:	22%
Lean mass:	91.2 lbs
Fat mass	26 lbs
Category:	Acceptable

Her total weight loss amounted to 8 lbs (just over half a stone) with body fat dropping by an impressive 6%. Although lean body mass only increased by 1.7 pounds – Pamela only managed to complete weight training once per week – she was able to switch her muscles into a positive nitrogen balance as a result of eating the right proteins and carbohydrates. Mobility was also increased thanks to an improved muscle tone.

Step 5 – Maintain

Life after the Nitro+ Diet

So, you've been following the Nitro+ Diet and working out with the Kinetic for four whole weeks. Now what? Well, life does go on, but that doesn't mean we leave all this stuff behind us. You've been making a big effort to reach your ideal weight and lean body mass, and I've no doubt that you'll have experienced a big change in your body and your relationship to it.

Remember, now, how I promised that your surplus fat was going to go, and go quickly? Even better, the Nitro+ Diet was designed so that body fat will stay away. You just need to make sure the Nitro+ Principles we've been establishing remain as a fixture in your lifestyle.

The Nitro+ Diet is the product of years of trial and error with my clients both at home and in the gym. Most clients want the same thing – to strip body fat, get leaner and improve their fitness. For some it's about looking good for an upcoming event such as a wedding or special party, or maybe something more athletic such as a triathlon or fun run. Yes, great results will be seen in as little as four weeks, but I do recommend sticking with it for as long as eight weeks. Let it become a way of life, so it sits comfortably with your normal routine.

- Stay away from fast food and high fat foods
- Keep well hydrated
- Don't eat late and avoid carbs after 8pm
- Continue with supplementation
- Maintain a PNB (Positive Nitrogen Balance)
- Always consume protein at breakfast

When you are happy with your new weight and Lean Body Mass, you'll be able to increase your carbohydrate intake to a level you're more comfortable with. Don't be surprised if this is less than you used to load onto your plate! You can reduce your protein levels a little, too, but please keep a watchful eye out for unnecessary fats – especially saturated fats, which are not at all good for you.

Coming up are some useful formulas to help you to calculate the ideal food intake levels to maintain your weight and continue fat loss. This is also known as your *LBM maintenance indicator*. Please note, there are separate calculations for men and for women.

If this seems like too much faff, don't worry, there is an easier way. Go to *www.bellmatesystems.com*, then click on the FREE Nitro+ Diet Calculator. Select "Nitro+ 7 site LBM maintenance calculator" from the dropdown menu and key in your age, new weight, gender, age and your 7 site measurements. Find out right away your new daily maintenance food requirements!

Women:

Calculate your new ideal food intake levels

- Work out your new Lean Body Mass (see Step 1 – Measure)
- Multiply your LBM by 0.7 to identify your New Protein Level
- Multiply this new protein level by 2.5 to identify New Carbohydrates Level
- Divide new protein level by 2.5 to indicate New Fat Level

For example:

Female LBM is now 100.

- To calculate recommended daily protein intake:
100 x 0.7 = 70 grams of protein per day
- To calculate recommended daily carbohydrates (low glycemic):
70 x 2.5 = 175 grams of carbohydrates per day
- To calculate recommended daily fats (unsaturated)
70 ÷ 2.5 = 28 grams of fats per day

The table filling the next couple of pages provides a useful guideline to help you figure out approximate nutritional intakes for different weights and LBMs. You'll need to get your fat measured so that you can work out your LBM maintenance indicator.

Note that the calculation for total calories is the result of multiplying figures for protein and carbohydrates by four, and fats by nine.

Nitro+ Maintenance Chart: Women

Weight (lbs)	Body fat %	Body fat (lbs)	LBM (lbs)	Protein (g)	Carbs (g)	Fats (g)	Calories
120	40	48	72	50	125	20	880
120	35	42	78	55	138	22	970
120	30	36	84	59	148	24	1044
120	25	30	90	63	158	25	1109
120	20	24	96	67	168	27	1183
130	40	52	78	55	138	22	970
130	35	46	84	59	148	24	1044
130	30	39	91	64	160	26	1130
130	25	33	97	68	170	27	1195
130	20	26	104	73	182.5	29	1283
140	40	56	84	59	148	24	1044
140	35	49	91	64	160	26	1130
140	30	42	98	69	173	28	1220
140	25	35	105	74	185	30	1306
140	20	28	112	78	195	31	1371
150	40	60	90	63	158	25	1109
150	35	53	97	68	170	27	1195
150	30	45	105	74	185	30	1306
150	25	38	112	78	195	31	1371
150	20	30	120	84	210	34	1482
160	40	64	96	67	168	27	1183
160	35	56	104	73	183	29	1285
160	30	48	112	78	195	31	1371
160	25	40	120	84	210	34	1482
160	20	32	128	90	225	36	1584
170	40	68	102	71	178	28	1248
170	35	59.5	111	77	193	31	1359
170	30	51	119	83	208	33	1461

The Nitro+ Diet

Weight (lbs)	Body fat %	Body fat (lbs)	LBM (lbs)	Protein (g)	Carbs (g)	Fats (g)	Calories
170	25	42.5	128	89	223	36	1572
170	20	34	136	95	238	38	1674
180	40	72	108	76	190	30	1334
180	35	63	117	82	205	33	1445
180	30	54	126	88	220	35	1547
180	25	45	135	94	236	38	1662
180	20	36	144	101	253	40	1776
190	40	76	114	80	200	32	1408
190	35	67	123	86	215	34	1510
190	30	57	133	93	234	37	1641
190	25	48	142	99	248	40	1748
190	20	38	152	106	265	42	1862
200	40	80	120	84	210	34	1482
200	35	70	130	91	228	36	1600
200	30	60	140	98	245	39	1723
200	25	50	150	105	263	42	1850
200	20	40	160	112	280	45	1973
210	40	84	126	88	220	35	1547
210	35	74	136	95	238	38	1674
210	30	63	147	103	258	41	1813
210	25	52	158	111	278	44	1952
210	20	42	168	118	295	47	2075
220	40	88	132	92	230	37	1621
220	35	77	143	100	250	40	1760
220	30	66	154	108	270	43	1899
220	25	55	165	116	290	46	2038
220	20	44	176	123	308	49	2165
230	40	92	138	97	243	39	1711
230	35	81	149	104	260	41	1825
230	30	69	161	113	283	45	1989

Weight (lbs)	Body fat %	Body fat (lbs)	LBM (lbs)	Protein (g)	Carbs (g)	Fats (g)	Calories
230	25	58	172	120	300	48	2112
230	20	46	184	129	323	52	2276
240	40	96	144	101	253	40	1776
240	35	84	156	109	273	44	1924
240	30	72	168	118	295	47	2075
240	25	60	180	126	315	50	2214
240	20	48	192	134	335	54	2362
250	40	100	150	105	263	42	1850
250	35	88	162	113	283	45	1989
250	30	75	175	123	308	49	2165
250	25	63	187	131	328	52	2304
250	20	50	200	140	350	56	2464

Men:
Calculate your new ideal food intake levels

- Work out your new Lean Body Mass (see Step 1 – Measure)
- Multiply your LBM by 0.9 to determine your New Protein Level
- Multiply this new protein level by 2.5 to identify New Carbohydrates Level
- Divide new protein level by 2.5 to find New Fat Level

For example:

Male LBM is now 150.

- To calculate recommended daily protein intake:
150 x 0.9 = 135 grams of protein per day

- To calculate recommended daily carbohydrates (low glycaemic):
135 x 2.5 = 337.5 grams of carbohydrates / day

- To calculate recommended daily fats (unsaturated)
135 ÷ 2.5 = 54 grams of fats per day

Nitro+ Maintenance Chart: Men

Weight (lbs)	Body fat %	Body fat (lbs)	LBM (lbs)	Protein (g)	Carbs (g)	Fats (g)	Calories
150	40	60	90	81	203	32	1424
150	35	52.5	98	88	221	35	1551
150	30	45	105	95	238	38	1674
150	25	38	113	102	255	41	1797
150	20	30	120	108	270	43.2	1900.8
160	40	64	96	86	215	34	1510
160	35	56	104	94	235	38	1658
160	30	48	112	101	253	40	1776
160	25	40	120	108	270	43	1899
160	20	32	128	115	288	46	2026
170	40	68	102	92	230	37	1621
170	35	59.5	111	100	250	40	1760
170	30	51	119	107	268	43	1887
170	25	43	128	115	288	46	2026
170	20	34	136	122	305	49	2149

Weight (lbs)	Body fat %	Body fat (lbs)	LBM (lbs)	Protein (g)	Carbs (g)	Fats (g)	Calories
180	40	72	108	97	243	39	1711
180	35	63	117	105	263	42	1850
180	30	54	126	113	283	45	1989
180	25	45	135	122	305	49	2149
180	20	36	144	130	325	52	2288
190	40	76	114	103	258	41	1813
190	35	67	123	111	277	44	1948
190	30	57	133	120	300	48	2112
190	25	48	143	128	320	51	2251
190	20	38	152	137	343	55	2415
200	40	80	120	108	270	43	1899
200	35	70	130	117	293	47	2063
200	30	60	140	126	315	50	2214
200	25	50	150	135	338	54	2378
200	20	40	160	144	360	58	2538
210	40	84	126	113	283	45	1989
210	35	74	137	123	308	49	2165
210	30	63	147	132	330	53	2325
210	25	53	157	141	353	56	2480
210	20	42	168	151	378	60	2656
220	40	88	132	119	298	48	2100
220	35	77	143	129	323	51	2267
220	30	66	154	139	348	56	2452
220	25	55	165	149	373	60	2628
220	20	44	176	158	395	63	2779
230	40	92	138	124	310	50	2186
230	35	81	149	134	335	53	2353
230	30	69	161	145	363	58	2554
230	25	58	172	155	388	62	2730
230	20	46	184	166	415	67	2927

Weight (lbs)	Body fat %	Body fat (lbs)	LBM (lbs)	Protein (g)	Carbs (g)	Fats (g)	Calories
240	40	96	144	130	325	52	2288
240	35	84	156	140	350	56	2464
240	30	72	168	151	378	60	2656
240	25	60	180	162	405	65	2853
240	20	48	192	173	433	69	3045
250	40	100	150	135	338	54	2378
250	35	88	162	146	365	58	2566
250	30	75	175	158	395	63	2779
250	25	63	187	168	420	67	2955
250	20	50	200	180	450	72	3168
260	40	104	156	140	350	56	2464
260	35	91	169	152	380	61	2677
260	30	78	182	164	410	66	2890
260	25	65	195	176	440	70	3094
260	20	52	208	187	468	75	3295
270	40	108	162	146	365	58	2566
270	35	95	175	158	395	63	2779
270	30	81	189	170	425	68	2992
270	25	68	202	182	455	73	3205
270	20	54	216	194	485	77	3409
280	40	112	168	151	378	60	2656
280	35	98	182	164	410	66	2890
280	30	84	196	176	440	70	3094
280	25	70	210	189	473	76	3332
280	20	56	224	202	505	81	3557

Calculating your ideal food intake levels will allow you to tailor the Nitro+ maintenance eating plan to your own needs. Stick with it, and the fat is sure to keep falling off.

Here's a reminder of some of the key principles that you should be following:

> - Drink warm lemon juice first thing in the morning
> - Consume a protein only breakfast
> - No carbohydrates after 8pm
> - Carry on taking chromium, zinc and L-carnitine on a daily basis
> - Take calcium & vitamin D supplement daily to keep the fat at bay
> - Keep taking CLA to keep the fat at bay
> - Consume 50% of your carbohydrates at lunch
> - Drink green tea
> - Stay hydrated
> - Sleep well

Keep the fat at bay

If you're someone who's done the rounds of all sorts of diets, you'll probably have noticed that as soon as the dieting period is over, the pounds start piling back on. Even worse, 75% of this resurgent weight is likely to be body fat! For every extra 10 lbs registering on the bathroom scales, 7.5 lbs will be fat. So maybe that celebratory cream cake wasn't such a good idea!

This sort of experience can be tremendously disheartening. You'll be feeling out of control, wondering why you went through all those weeks of denial and discipline. But there is another way – the Nitro+ way.

We can stop the fat from accumulating again, by staying in control of our lifestyle. The most important thing is to maintain a positive nitrogen balance by consuming protein foods throughout the day. Avoid consuming any carbohydrates after 8pm and carry on taking the supplements.

CLA

Conjugated linoleic acid reduces body fat by increasing the basal metabolic rate. While it doesn't do much to decrease overall body weight, it can prevent those little fat cells from getting any bigger. This is much more important as it can improve the fat / muscle ratio.

A comparative study of people in the aftermath of following a diet revealed some interesting results. Those who stopped dieting without maintaining CLA status sure enough put weight back on – at the worrying proportion of 75% fat to 25% muscle. A second group of participants continued to take CLA; although they also gained weight, this was at the far more healthy ratio of 50% fat, 50% muscle.

So, even though the Nitro+ Diet is designed to last at most 8 weeks at a time, it's not going to leave you in the lurch. Your body fat is going to drop off, and with the help of supplements as part of your maintenance regime, it is going to stay off.

Magnesium

Magnesium plays its part in fat loss and makes the cell receptors more receptive to insulin. It will also help you sleep. Magnesium complements the effects of calcium on obesity and when taken together with calcium and vitamin D can crank up your fat burning engine by a whole extra gear.

Vitamin D

This vitamin is fantastic for directly burning body fat and will also reduce the amount of enzymes responsible for fat storage. It's a big help in keeping your fat burning switch turned on.

Calcium

Calcium's public image – largely thanks to the efforts of the Milk Marketing Board – is all about building up bone structure, so you may be surprised to learn that it can also be a big help in promoting weight loss.

A recent comparative study demonstrated that increased amounts of calcium in the diet can have significant effects on fat loss. How did they find this out? They measured the fat content of poo – faecal fat, in technical terms, which is an indicator of how well your liver, gallbladder, pancreas and intestines are working. Maybe you find this a bit gross, but it amounted to losing an extra 350 calories a day. And that's something not to be sniffed at!

This is by no means the only study indicating that calcium plays an important role in fat metabolism. It's evidently going to be a useful ally in your quest to decrease weight and body fat, particularly when you're on the rebound from a diet regime.

> ### *Nitro+ Principle # 23*
> ## Take calcium, magnesium & vitamin D supplement to cut fat cells down to size

Stay hydrated

Water, like nitrogen, is everywhere, a crucial part of the dance of life. By far the most of this water is salty, held in the oceans which cover 71% of our planet's surface. A mere 3.5% of the total quantity is fresh water, either flowing through the world's lake and river systems or locked away in the Earth's freezer compartment, the glaciers and polar ice caps.

It's a big part of who we are, too. Men have around 60% water in their bodies and women have around 55%. It does all sorts of jobs for us, including removing waste, regulating body temperature, and lubricating joints. From our particular point of view, it's also a fantastic natural appetite suppressant and metabolic facilitator.

In short, the consumption of water is vital to the normal functioning of the body. You could survive for days, weeks, even months with scarcely any food, but just two or three days without water is going to prove fatal.

Scientists define dehydration as fluid losses greater than 1% of your bodyweight. A loss of 5% bodyweight through dehydration has been shown to produce approximately a 30% decrease in performance. Optimal body function depends on keeping up the water level. Water comprises around 75% of muscle whereas in fat there's a mere 10-15%. Athletes take special care to stay well hydrated, and so should you – if you're dehydrated, it's going to be difficult to burn body fat.

Dehydration has many symptoms, depending on the severity of the condition. The table below offers a guide, with particular reference to infants and children.

Mild to moderate dehydration

• Dry, sticky mouth	• Thirst
• Decreased urine output	• Dry skin
• Dry skin	• Headache
• Fatigue	• Dizziness
• Few or no tears	• Constipation
• Sleepiness or tiredness — children are likely to be less active than usual	
• In infants, no wet nappies for three hours	

Severe dehydration

- Extreme fussiness or sleepiness in infants and children; irritability and confusion in adults
- Very dry mouth, skin and mucous membranes
- Little or no urination — any urine that is produced will be darker than normal
- Shrivelled and dry skin that lacks elasticity and doesn't 'bounce back' when pinched into a fold
- In infants, sunken fontanels — the soft spots on the top of a baby's head

• Sunken eyes	• No tears when crying
• Low blood pressure	• Rapid breathing
• Rapid heartbeat	• Fever

Urine Check

Checking your hydration level is easily done: simply pay attention to the colour of your urine. As I'm sure you've noticed, it doesn't always look the same; it's telling you something valuable about your current state, so it's worth some serious consideration.

- *Pale yellow*

  Watery, pale yellow urine with little odour is a good sign that all is well from a hydration point of view. Remember, when we are well hydrated we burn more body fat.

- *Dark yellow*

  This is the sort of outcome you may well have experienced the morning after a boozy session with your mates. It's an indicator of mild dehydration, following the body's best efforts to rid itself of all that intoxicating liquor, and it's going to be a bit on the smelly side. You'd be well off drinking a couple of glasses of water to top up your fluid levels.

  If dehydration doesn't seem to be the obvious cause, do consider that there might be an underlying medical cause, such as hepatitis, anaemia or haematuria. It's certainly worth consulting a doctor about.

- *Green*

  Unless you happen to be the Incredible Hulk or an alien from the planet Zog, this may be a consequence of some medications (such as rinsapin), artificial food colourings or simply the asparagus you ate last night.

- *Blue*

  No, I'm not taking the piss – this could indeed happen!

It's not very common, though, and most likely would be caused by medication containing pteridine.

- **Pink**

  All girls would love to have pink urine that has an odour like flowers – right? Eating beetroot would certainly produce the desired colour, if not the smell – there's even a special name for this (beeturia). Don't mistake this, in any case, for blood in the urine (haematuria), which is a definite cause for concern. Most likely it's not a sign of anything life-threatening, but it could be indicative of problems with kidneys, bladder, prostate or urethra. Make an appointment with your doctor.

- **Orange**

  "What's up, Doc?" Orange urine could be the result of eating lots of carrots or foods high in beta-carotene. It can also indicate dehydration or possible jaundice.

Nitro+ Principle # 24
Stay well hydrated

You know those times when you're desperate to eat something – anything! – right now . . . well, it could be that what you really need is something to drink. Some interesting research has been done on the connections between hydration and obesity.

A study conducted at the University of Washington demonstrated that drinking just one 8 oz glass of water eliminated hunger pangs in 98% of the subjects. Moreover, the Journal of Clinical Endocrinology and

Metabolism (2003) reported that consuming 16 oz (two glasses) of water resulted in a 30% increase in metabolic rate, largely attributable to the energy expenditure required to warm the water to normal body temperature.

If you think you may be dehydrated, you already are. Remember to keep drinking plenty of fluids throughout the day, but not while you're eating.

You might be surprised at how much fluid your body requires each day to stay functioning at its most efficient. Here's a chart which breaks it all down, in terms of cupfuls – equivalent to 200 ml (approximately 8 fl oz).

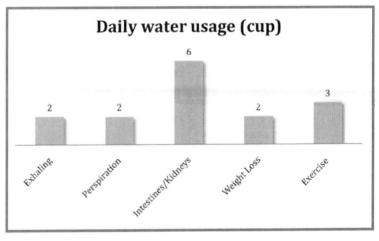

Each day, two cups of water are exhaled when we breathe, two cups are lost through sweating and a further two cups are needed to enable weight loss. Healthy functioning of the intestines and kidneys – the processes of digestion and excretion – requires a further six cups per day. If you're going to be exercising you should add another three cups. So that's a total of 12 cups a day, or

15 on training days. That's a lot of water!

Hydration is crucial both for maintaining general health and for losing body fat. If you are dehydrated your fat burning switch will be turned off. Staying well hydrated will switch the fat burning engine on as well as helping you to stave off food cravings and remain focussed.

Now, pass me that water bottle . . .

www.livestrong.com
www.nutrition411.com/content/fluid-requirements-adults

Sleeping burns body fat

Well, this looks like good news! Seems like all I need to do is go to sleep and I will lose body fat! Have I got this right?

Unfortunately, it's not quite that straightforward. The benefits of getting a good night's sleep are of course manifold, while sleep deprivation can cause chaos on both physical and mental levels. We're going to take a brief look at how the quality and quantity of your shuteye can impact on your metabolism.

When we sleep well we have a reduced cortisol level. Cortisol is a steroid hormone with an impact on blood glucose production which varies according to the degree of fasting. Normally, the quantity of cortisol in the body follows a daily rhythm: after bottoming out in the wee small hours it hits a peak just around breakfast time, just in time to pack away excess glycogen into the liver. Not sleeping throws a real spanner in the works, increasing glucose and insulin sensitivity, reducing your energy levels and kickstarting carbohydrate cravings. It's the last thing you need when you're trying to cut down on calories.

Too much cortisol bouncing around in the body can result in breakdown of muscle tissue and put you into an unwanted catabolic state. Reducing calories and going on a diet can increase cortisol levels, but as long as you keep to the Nitro+ Diet protein levels you'll be able to keep muscle breakdown under control.

Sleep is very important. When we sleep we go into different phases in two zones. The first is called non- REM sleep. REM stands for rapid eye movement.

Non-REM Zone

• Stage 1

Going to sleep: the stage where you've shut your eyes but could easily come back awake. It lasts for around 10-15 minutes, though if you have a lot of thoughts swirling round your mind this stage may last a little longer. Try to relax and empty your thoughts.

• Stage 2

Very light sleep, as your body readies itself for deeper sleep. At this point your body temperature starts to drop and your heart rate slows. You will find it harder to wake.

• Stage 3

This is when we enter deep sleep. It's harder to wake up and if we are woken we feel groggy, as if we've been drugged. The body is busy, though, with the business of rejuvenation: hormone production peaks, allowing the immune system to restore itself.

REM Zone

- **Stage 4**

Around 90 minutes after the onset of sleep, heart rate and breathing start to increase, almost as if we are coming awake. Deep sleep gives way to the rapid eye movement stage, in which most of our muscles are immobilised while the brain gets busy with all sorts of things – the stuff of dreams.

The function of dreaming remains mysterious, but it evidently it plays an important role in processing our waking experiences. Babies can spend up to 50% of their sleep in the REM zone compared to only 20% in adults.

Exercise, Nutrition & Rest – a three way split

Sleep allows the body to repair itself, to restore effective functionality. It's not something we should compromise on. I like to remember the health equation: which is the most important, exercise, nutrition, or rest?

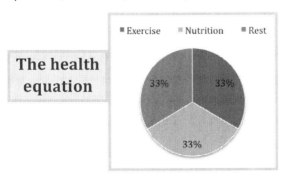

The health equation

I expect you guessed what I'm going to say: they're

each as important as each other – an exact three way split. When you get all of these right everything becomes possible – you can easily strip body fat, build muscle and reach your goal. Don't underestimate the power of rest, it's just as important as proper nutrition and healthy exercise. If you wake up one morning and don't feel up to the gym, don't go. Listen to your body, maybe it's saying you need to rest. In which case, the best thing you can do may well be to skip the workout and go fix yourself up with some carbohydrates.

A recent study reported in the American Journal of Clinical Nutrition found that when people had little sleep they experienced more cravings for late night high carbohydrate snacks. Another study demonstrated that inadequate sleep correlated with larger portion sizes and increased high carbohydrate bingeing.

So, the bottom line is, get enough sleep, preferably in a dark quiet room. When we sleep well we think and perform better.

Exercise + Nutrition + Rest = the Results You Want

Nitro+ Principle # 25
Get 7-8 hours of quality sleep every night

Alcohol

There's no point being holier than thou here, I've got to admit that I enjoy the odd glass of crispy white, or relaxing with a pint of beer. I know I'm not the only one – it's a defining part of our culture. And the question keeps coming up when I speak to people about nutrition:

"Can I drink alcohol on this diet?"

It's as if our lives depend on it; it's certainly a big factor in people's reasoning whether they should give the Nitro+ Diet a go. Well . . . I do understand it could be difficult if alcohol plays a significant role in your daily agenda of meetings and greetings, lubricating the wheels of business with a sociable shared bevvy or two. Peer group pressure, the urge to fit in, can become an issue.

But . . . facts are facts: alcohol is a poison. It slowly corrupts the body, even while it dissolves inhibitions and releases mental straightjackets. Many people ask me about the calories in alcohol and whether it's better sticking to spirits. The problem is not so much with the calories but what it actually does to the body. It's like putting the wrong fuel in your car – your car won't like it and it will not work very well . . . just cough, splutter and conk out! Don't believe me? Give a moment to consider some of the ways in which alcohol can harm the body:

- **Brain:** it can interfere with the brain's communication pathway and affect mood and behaviour.
- **Heart:** alcohol can cause the heart to stretch and droop (cardiomyopathy), develop an irregular heart-beat and increase the chances of stroke and high blood pressure. It should be noted, however, that there is research out there suggesting that drinking moderate amounts of alcohol may help protect you from developing coronary heart disease.

- **Pancreas:** alcohol can make the pancreas produce toxic substances leading to pancreatitis (inflammation of blood vessels preventing proper digestion).
- **Liver:** we all know that drinking affects the liver. It can lead to a variety of problems such as fatty liver, fibrosis, cirrhosis and alcoholic hepatitis.
- **Cancer:** drinking too much alcohol can increase the risk of developing cancers such as mouth, breast, throat, liver and oesophageal cancer.
- **Immune system:** your immune system will be compromised if you drink too much alcohol and you are more likely to develop tuberculosis and pneumonia.

www.niaaa.nih.gov/alcohol-health/alcohols-effects-body

Alcohol and Obesity

As if all that wasn't enough bad news, alcohol makes you fat. Just a few drinks can interfere with the normal sleep cycle, knocking you into deep sleep without the benefits of REM, which normally occurs 6-7 times during the night. It'll leave you feeling tired in the morning, as if you've missed out on something important.

Another problem with alcohol is the dehydration that follows on from flushing out the toxins from the body. It also makes you snore loudly, act like a twerp, do things you're going to regret tomorrow . . . not to mention giving you a stonking headache.

Here's my advice: give your wife, husband, kids, liver, and bank balance a break – drop the alcohol.

> ### *Nitro+ Principle # 26*
> ## Knock the booze on the head

Overtraining

When we are sleep deprived but exercising regularly we can push things too far – we can overtrain. This is due to suppression of the immune system and lack of rest. Signs of overtraining are increased waking heart rate, reduction in bodyweight and insomnia (difficulty in sleeping). If you feel that you are heading into the overtraining zone stop training for one week, increase carbohydrates to 70% of total calories, drop the protein to 15% of total calories, boost antioxidants and increase your sleep to nine hours per night.

For most adults the optimal level of uninterrupted sleep is 7-8 hours. This will give your body and mind the rest that it needs to recover from the day, as well as being very important for fat loss.

So what have we learned?

Congratulations on sticking with this book all the way through. I do hope you've enjoyed reading it, but more importantly I hope I've persuaded you to give the Nitro+ Diet your full attention, dedication and resolve. You won't regret it.

I recommend that you try the diet, together with the exercise regime, for four to eight weeks. After four weeks you'll already be seeing fantastic results. I know, because I've followed it myself many times, and it has always been successful.

Use the Nitro+ system as a tool, to be used as and when you need it. This is what marks it out from most traditional and faddy diets. When you've achieved your optimum weight and LBM, feel free to ease up . . . you can always pick things up again if that seems necessary, but my guess is you'll have learnt enough about how your body works, and how to manage your metabolism, to avoid slipping back into those old fat-building habits. You'll have managed to transform your relationship with your body.

The reason it works is that it's all about creating an anabolic environment which encourages muscle retention. It's not simply about losing weight – you'll be losing fat, rather than muscle. And that's what makes it distinct from so many other diets, which achieve their results largely by losing water and muscle tissue. When you ease up on those diets, the body goes into survival mode, locking away fats and carbohydrates just in case famine ever kicks in again. In many cases you can end up heavier than when you started! No wonder these are known as yo-yo diets.

The Nitro+ Diet is all about empowerment. You'll have learnt what to eat, and when. You'll have the ignition keys for your internal fat furnace. And you'll be armed with a set of basic principles to keep you trim, the size and shape you want to be.

I would love to hear from you and how the Nitro+ Diet has changed your life. Please click on to our website – *www.bellmatesystems.com* – and share your experience. Post some pictures. Become part of the Kinetic revolution.

Ok, so what happens now? Check back through the book if you like, reread those bits you maybe didn't quite get first time round, and make a note of the principles, somewhere handy like on your mobile phone. They'll be a sort of condensed operating manual. And you'll be in the driver's seat.

You can achieve anything if you put your mind to it. Believe in yourself, visualise how you want to look, stay focussed, be disciplined, go out there and JUST DO IT!

Oh . . . and Good Luck.

That's enough from me . . . now it's over to you – become part of the Kinetic Revolution!

Case Study # 6 – John

Our final case study concerns John, a 65 year old man. John had difficulties with excess body fat around the tummy, but his main issue was muscle wastage (negative nitrogen balance), together with a poor diet and the onset of arthritis.

The Nitro+ Diet was introduced, kicking off with a four day detox plan. He began weight training three or four times per week, three sets with a rep range of 8-10. The main aim was to switch the muscles back into positive nitrogen balance, enabling body fat to be utilised for energy, improving general health and mobility and encouraging both fat loss and muscle growth.

Before Nitro+ training	
Start weight:	142 lbs
Body fat %-age:	30%
Lean mass:	99 lbs
Fat mass:	43 lbs
Category:	Overweight
After four weeks	
Weight:	136 lbs
Body fat %-age:	27%
Lean mass:	99 lbs
Fat mass:	37 lbs
Category:	Acceptable

John felt deservedly happy with the result: a fat loss of 6 pounds, with joints a lot less inflamed. The lean muscle remained the same – at his age muscle is harder to build – but if he were to keep up with this regime for a further four weeks there's no doubt muscle growth would commence, while fat would continue to be stripped away.

Appendix A
Some recipe ideas

How do you like your eggs?

Eggs are such a great way of boosting your protein intake, so here's a selection of preparation strategies, kicking off with the basic quick fix, then stretching out into more adventurous territory.

Scrambled Eggs

This is one my favourite breakfast dishes. It's fast, healthy and anyone can cook it – even me. It wastes no time in kicking the body into the fat burning zone.

Ingredients
- 2-3 large British Lion eggs
- 30 ml / 2 Tbs milk
- Salt and freshly ground black pepper

Method
You can use a microwave for this, which makes it a lot easier to prepare and just as effective (though you might have qualms about the micro-radiation).

Crack two or three eggs into a microwave-proof bowl or jug. If you want to reduce the amount of cholesterol, remove one or two of the yolks. Add the milk, season with salt or pepper, and whisk it all together until well mixed.

I normally allow 30 seconds per egg depending on the microwave setting. Give it a whisk, or a swirl with the fork, every 20 seconds until the eggs are suitably scrambled. Don't leave in for too long as they may overcook and dry out, and bear in mind that the eggs will still be cooking when you remove them from the microwave, so make allowances for this.

Egg Surprise

This is really one of my own recipes and I have named it Egg Surprise. It's basically the same as the scrambled eggs with added smoked salmon!

Ingredients
- 2-3 large British Lion eggs
- 30 ml / 2 Tbs milk
- Salt and freshly ground black pepper
- Smoked salmon

Method
Follow the same procedure as above, but have the surprise ingredient – some smoked salmon cut into squares – ready for adding to the scramble. It really is simple as that!

Omelette aux Fines Herbes

There are of course all sorts of ways to take advantage of the high quality protein packed into a humble egg. How about a classic omelette aux fines herbes? If you have fresh herbs growing in your garden, then this is a brilliant way to incorporate home produce into your diet.

Ideally, you'll need a heavy bottomed frying pan. For one or two portions, this should be around 9" diameter.

Allow two medium or large eggs per person. Whisk them up in a jug, and add a selection of finely cooked herbs according to choice. Parsley is always good, chives too; other good combinations are parsley and garlic, parsley and oregano . . . the possibilities are endless really. If you don't have fresh herbs to hand, then reach for the Italian dried herb mix. Sometimes I've even used chillies, for an added kick (though do be careful!). Add a bit of salt and pepper, plus a splash of water, and whisk well.

Heat a small amount of butter in the frying pan, so it spreads all over the base – this will prevent the omelette from sticking to the pan. Pour in the mix and heat gently. When the eggs are more or less set you can carefully (using a spatula) fold the omelette over to achieve a neat half moon shape.

Serve warm with a mixed salad as a lunch or dinner or, as a quick breakfast, on its own.

Frittata

You could say this is basically a thick omelette with more vegetable filling. There's an almost infinite range of possibilities to experiment with. There is also a choice between making this in an omelette pan, on the oven top, or in a casserole dish in the oven. If you opt for the latter, you'd be less likely to burn the bottom before the mixture is cooked through – especially if, like myself, you like to have a good thick, sliceable frittata.

Start by preparing your vegetables – onions, peppers, courgettes, aubergines, garlic . . . the choice is yours – cutting them to an even size. Heat a little butter in the pan and sauté for five to ten minutes to soften them up.

Mix up the eggs as with the omelette, then add the prepared vegetables and pour back into the frying pan. Heat gently until set, taking care not to burn the bottom. If you wish, you can add a little bit of grated cheese on top, which can be gently browned under a grill.

Serve up for dinner with a large salad. If you've made a lot, keep some by for a cold snack or brunch.

This dish is packed with protein, healthy fats and loads of vitamin A, C and K plus plenty of fibre.

Mini Smoked Salmon Frittatas

These are my personal favourites. They're packed with protein, plus omega-3 fatty acids, and very low in carbohydrates. So what are you waiting for?

This recipe makes six servings.

Ingredients

- 1 tablespoon extra virgin olive oil
- ¼ cup diced onion
- 6 large eggs
- 8 large egg whites
- 4 Tbs whole milk
- ½ tsp salt
- freshly ground black pepper
- 3 oz reduced fat cream cheese, cubed
- 4 oz smoked salmon, cut into ¼ inch pieces
- 2 Tbs spring onions, thinly sliced, for garnish

Method

Preheat the oven to 325°F, 170°C (gas Mk 3). Chop the onions, then gently heat the oil in a skillet, and sauté the onions for a few minutes until soft. Allow to cool.

Measure the eggs into a bowl, and whisk together with the milk and seasoning. Stir in the cream cheese. Add the onions.

Prepare 6 (8 oz) ramekins by lightly coating bottom and sides with oil or butter. Add 2 Tbs of smoked salmon to each ramekin, then pour ¾ cup of egg mixture on top, being careful not to overfill.

Place the ramekins on a baking sheet, then bake for 25 minutes, or until a wooden pick inserted into the centre comes out clean.

Serve garnished with spring onions.

Nutritional Information	
Calories per serving:	179
Fat per serving:	11 g
Protein per serving:	17 g
Carbohydrate per serving:	3 g
Fibre per serving:	0.0 g

Based on myrecipes.com

Cheesy Cast-Iron Skillet Scrambled Eggs

This is another one of my favourites. It's a sort of scrambled eggs deluxe, with an extra protein fix from the added cheese. There's a few extra minutes involved in the preparation – 10-12 minutes, say – but if this is what it takes to head into the realm of gastronomic delight, who's complaining?

As the name suggests, you'll need a largish cast iron skillet – a heavy-bottomed frying pan, in other words. You'll notice that the recipe features jalapeño pepper, which can vary considerably in spiciness. My advice: use ingredients you are familiar with.

The quantities overleaf will do for two or three portions.

Ingredients

- 1 Tbs unsalted butter
- ½ small red onion, finely diced
- ½ jalapeño pepper, sliced in thin rounds
- 6 large eggs, lightly beaten
- salt & freshly ground black pepper to taste
- 2 oz (60 g) goat cheese, crumbled
- 1 Tbs finely chopped chives

Method

Melt the butter in a large-ish cast iron skillet over a medium flame. Add onion and jalapeño and cook until soft (5-7 minutes). Stir in eggs, salt and pepper, then cook, stirring constantly, until soft curds form (about 3 minutes).

Remove skillet from the heat and fold in the goat cheese and chives. Serve immediately with whole-grain toast or English muffin, if desired.

Spinach & Egg Wrap with Avocado, Pepper & Cheese

It's a wrap! – packed with protein, loaded with magnesium, potassium and Vitamin B6, and guaranteed to look after your heart. This is another recipe derived from *myrecipes.com*, to serve two portions.

Ingredients

- Nonstick cooking spray
- 70 g baby spinach, chopped
- 2 eggs
- 2 egg whites
- salt & freshly ground black pepper to taste
- 2 oz grated cheddar cheese
- 1 avocado, sliced
- 2 whole-wheat tortillas
- Hot sauce

Method

For minimal fat content, spray a non-stick skillet and heat over a medium flame. If you don't have this spray in your cupboard, then you can use a little olive oil. Add spinach and cook, stirring, until wilted – about two minutes.

Whisk together eggs and egg whites in a small bowl. Add eggs to the skillet and cook, stirring, until curds form – a couple of minutes. Season with salt and pepper.

Place half of the egg mixture in the centre of each tortilla, and sprinkle with the grated cheese.

Top with slices of avocado and fold, burrito-style. Slice in half and serve, with a side order of spicy sauce.

Nutritional Information	
Calories per serving:	366
Fat per serving:	22 g
Protein per serving:	22 g
Carbohydrate per serving:	30 g
Fibre per serving:	7 g

Asparagus with Poached Eggs & Parmesan

Here's another recipe derived from *myrecipes.com*. It's an exciting combo ideal for breakfast or lunch. Asparagus is fantastic for keeping your cardiovascular system in shape and will provide you with extra energy for the day.

This recipe is for two servings, a real pleasure to share.

Ingredients

- 4 large eggs
- ½ tsp white vinegar
- ½ tsp salt, divided
- 1 bunch asparagus spears, trimmed (about 20)
- ½ Tbs extra-virgin olive oil
- 1 garlic clove, chopped
- 1 Tbs butter
- 1 Tbs fresh lemon juice
- 1 tsp finely chopped fresh parsley
- Freshly ground black pepper, to taste
- 2 Tbs coarsely grated fresh parmesan cheese

Method

Break the eggs carefully into four individual containers (such as teacups, prep bowls, or paper cups). Fill a medium saucepan with water, add the vinegar and half of the salt, then bring to a rolling boil.

Meanwhile, prepare the asparagus. To remove any woodiness, snap each spear and discard the bottom end. Heat another medium pan of water to boiling, add the asparagus and cook for about four minutes, until crisply tender. Remove asparagus with tongs, plunge into cold water for a couple of minutes, then drain.

Dry your saucepan, add olive oil, and heat over a medium flame. Add garlic, and sauté for about a minute. Turn off the heat, add butter, and swirl the ingredients in the pan. Add lemon juice, parsley, and seasoning; swirl the pan again to combine. Add asparagus and half the parmesan, then toss together with the lemon-butter sauce until well coated.

Slowly and carefully pour each egg into the boiling poaching water; cook for two minutes (use a timer!). Meanwhile, get ready to serve up. Divide the asparagus between two serving plates and place next to the egg pan, with a folded kitchen towel laid out handy.

Turn off the heat, and remove the eggs from the water using a slotted spoon. Make use of the kitchen towel to soak up any loose water, then place two eggs on each mound of asparagus. Pour any remaining sauce over each serving, and sprinkle with the rest of the parmesan. Serve immediately.

Nutritional Information	
Calories per serving:	256
Fat per serving:	11 g
Protein per serving:	18 g
Carbohydrate per serving:	8 g
Fibre per serving:	3 g

Fruit Smoothie with Soy Milk

Very refreshing, particularly when you're after something cool and delicious. Makes four servings.

Ingredients

- 3 cups (600 ml) plain or vanilla soy milk
- 1 banana, peeled, chopped and frozen
- 1 cup frozen strawberries or raspberries
- A few drops vanilla or almond extract

Method

You'll need to have thought about this in advance, making sure you have some fruit in the freezer, maybe in portion-sized bags. When you feel smitten by that smoothie moment, you can load up blender or food processor and give it a whizz until smooth and tasty.

Appendix B
Your Nitro+ Principles

Nitro+ Principle # 1
Forget all other diets that focus on weight loss

Nitro+ Principle # 2
Avoid high sugar fruit juices, fizzy drinks & diet drinks

Nitro+ Principle # 3
Avoid Aspartame sweetener

Nitro+ Principle # 4
Avoid Starchy Foods

Nitro+ Principle # 5
Drink warm water with fresh lemon juice upon rising, before breakfast

Nitro+ Principle # 6
Lunch like a prince and dine like a pauper

Nitro+ Principle # 7
Stick to polyunsaturated and mono-unsaturated fats

Nitro+ Principle # 8
Eat a protein only breakfast

Nitro+ Principle # 9

Consume protein within one hour of finishing training, together with some simple carbohydrates for anti-catabolism

Nitro+ Principle # 10

Snack between meals on fruit, nuts and seeds

Nitro+ Principle # 11

Consume 35% of your low GL carbohydrates at lunch

Nitro+ Principle # 12

Consume 30-50 grams of fibre per day

Nitro+ Principle # 13

Eat your proteins before your carbohydrates and don't drink fluids with your meal

Nitro+ Principle # 14

Reduce consumption of red and processed meats

Nitro+ Principle # 15

Consume NO carbohydrates after 8 pm

Nitro+ Principle # 16

Maintain daily recommended intake of chromium, zinc, and fish oil

Nitro+ Principle # 17

Consume 500 mg–1000 mg L-carnitine daily

Nitro+ Principle # 18
Drink 2-3 cups of green tea daily (or equivalent supplement) to boost your metabolism

Nitro+ Principle # 19
Crank up your metabolism with caffeine

Nitro+ Principle # 20
Consume CLA to burn fat and to stop it coming back

Nitro+ Principle # 21
Introduce resistance training 3 times per week, with small cardio intervals

Nitro+ Principle # 22
Train 3 times per week with the Kinetic to ignite your muscles

Nitro+ Principle # 23
Take calcium, magnesium and vitamin D supplement to cut fat cells down to size

Nitro+ Principle # 24
Stay well hydrated

Nitro+ Principle # 25
Get 7-8 hours of quality sleep every night

Nitro+ Principle # 26
Knock the booze on the head

Appendix C
Supplement Contraindications

This information is derived from *www.webmd.com*.

I recommend that, when taking supplements which affect the metabolism of your body, you do so as consciously as possible. Using diet supplements is optional; please read the following guide carefully so you can feel confident you're doing the right thing when you're lining up your daily supplements. Of course, if, having studied this information, you think something doesn't seem right, then do hold back and seek the advice of your doctor.

Chromium

Chromium is **LIKELY SAFE** for most adults when taken by mouth in doses up to 1000 mcg daily for up to 6 months. Chromium is **POSSIBLY SAFE** for most adults when used for longer periods of time. Some people experience side effects such as skin irritation, headaches, dizziness, mood changes, nausea, and impairment in thinking, judgment, and coordination. High doses have been linked to more serious side effects including blood disorders, liver or kidney damage and other problems. It is not known for sure if chromium is the actual cause of these side effects.

In children, chromium is **LIKELY SAFE** when taken by mouth in amounts that do not exceed the 'adequate intake' (AI) levels. Taking chromium by mouth is **POSSIBLY SAFE** when used in amounts that exceed the AI levels.

Special precautions & warnings:

Pregnancy and breast-feeding: Chromium is **LIKELY SAFE** to use during pregnancy and breast-feeding when taken by mouth in amounts that are equal to or less than 'adequate intake' (AI) levels. Chromium is **POSSIBLY SAFE** to use during pregnancy in amounts higher than the AI levels. However, pregnant women should not take chromium supplements during pregnancy or breast-feeding unless advised to do so by their healthcare provider.

Kidney disease: There are at least three reports of kidney damage in patients who took chromium picolinate. Don't take chromium supplements if you already have kidney disease.

Liver disease: There have been several reports of liver damage in patients who took chromium picolinate. Don't take chromium supplements if you already have liver disease.

Diabetes: Chromium might lower blood sugar levels too much if taken along with diabetes medications. If you have diabetes, use chromium products cautiously and monitor blood glucose levels closely. Dose adjustments to diabetes medications might be necessary.

Insulin interacts with chromium. Chromium might decrease blood sugar. Insulin is also used to decrease blood sugar. Taking chromium along with insulin might cause your blood sugar to be too low. Monitor your blood sugar closely. The dose of your insulin might need to be changed.

Behavioural or psychiatric conditions such as anxiety, depression, or schizophrenia: Chromium might affect brain chemistry and might make behavioural or psychiatric conditions worse. If you have one of these conditions, be careful when using chromium supplements. Pay attention to any changes in how you feel.

Chromate / leather contact allergy: Chromium supplements can cause allergic reactions in people with chromate or leather contact allergy. Symptoms include redness, swelling, and scaling of the skin.

Levothyroxine (Synthroid) interacts with chromium. Taking chromium with levothyroxine might decrease how much levothyroxine that the body absorbs. This might make levothyroxine less effective. To help avoid this interaction, levothyroxine should be taken 30 minutes before or 3-4 hours after taking chromium.

NSAIDs (non-steroidal anti-inflammatory drugs) interact with chromium. NSAIDs are anti-inflammatory medications used for decreasing pain and swelling. They might increase chromium levels in the body and increase the risk of adverse effects. Avoid taking chromium supplements and NSAIDs at the same time.

Examples of NSAIDs include ibuprofen (Advil, Motrin, Nuprin, others), indomethacin (Indocin), naproxen (Aleve, Anaprox, Naprelan, Naprosyn), piroxicam (Feldene), aspirin, and others.

L- Carnitine

L-carnitine is **LIKELY SAFE** for most people when taken by mouth and when used as an injection, with the approval of a healthcare provider. It can cause side effects such as nausea, vomiting, stomach upset, heartburn, diarrhea, and seizures. It can also cause the urine, breath, and sweat to have a 'fishy' odour.

Special precautions & warnings:

Pregnancy and breast-feeding: There is not enough reliable information about the safety of using L-carnitine if you are pregnant. Stay on the safe side and avoid use.

Taking L-carnitine is **POSSIBLY SAFE** in breast-feeding women when taken by mouth in the amounts recommended. Small amounts of L-carnitine have been given to infants in breast milk and formula with no reported side effects. The effects of large amounts taken by a breast-feeding mother are unknown.

Children: L-carnitine is **POSSIBLY SAFE** when used appropriately by mouth or intravenously (by IV), short-term.

Under-active thyroid (hypothyroidism): Taking L-carnitine might make symptoms of hypothyroidism worse.

Kidney failure: Using D-carnitine (an alternative form of carnitine, spiralling right rather than left) has been reported to cause symptoms such as muscle weakness and eye drooping when administered intravenously (by IV) after dialysis. L-carnitine does not seem to have this effect.

Seizures: L-carnitine seems to make seizures more likely in people who have had seizures before. If you have had a seizure, do not use L-carnitine.

Acenocoumarol (Sintrom) interacts with L-carnitine. This agent is used to slow blood clotting; L-carnitine might increase its effectiveness, perhaps by more than you reckoned on. You should consider changing your dose of acenocoumarol (Sintrom).

Thyroid hormone interacts with L-carnitine, which seems to reduce the effectiveness of thyroid hormone in the body

Warfarin (Coumadin), which is used to slow blood clotting, interacts with L-carnitine. L-carnitine might increase the effects of warfarin (Coumadin) and increase the chances of bruising and bleeding. Be sure to have your blood checked regularly. The dose of your warfarin (Coumadin) might need to be changed.

Zinc

Zinc is **LIKELY SAFE** for most adults when applied to the skin, or when taken by mouth in amounts not larger than 40 mg daily. Routine zinc supplementation is not recommended without the advice of a healthcare professional. In some people, zinc might cause nausea, vomiting, diarrhoea, metallic taste, kidney and stomach damage, and other side effects. Using zinc on broken skin may cause burning, stinging, itching, and tingling.

Zinc is **POSSIBLY SAFE** when taken by mouth in doses greater than 40 mg daily. There is some concern that taking doses higher than this might decrease how much copper the body absorbs. Decreased copper absorption may cause anaemia.

Zinc is **POSSIBLY UNSAFE** when inhaled through the nose, as it might cause permanent loss of smell. In June 2009, the US Food and Drug Administration (FDA) advised consumers not to use certain zinc-containing nose sprays (Zicam) after receiving over 100 reports of loss of smell. The maker of these zinc-containing nose sprays has also received several hundred reports of loss of smell from people who had used the products. Avoid using nose sprays containing zinc.

Taking high amounts of zinc is **LIKELY UNSAFE**. High doses above the recommended amounts might cause fever, coughing, stomach pain, fatigue, and many other problems.

Taking more than 100 mg of supplemental zinc daily or

taking supplemental zinc for 10 or more years doubles the risk of developing prostate cancer. There is also concern that taking large amounts of a multivitamin plus a separate zinc supplement increases the chance of dying from prostate cancer.

Taking 450 mg or more of zinc daily can cause problems with blood iron. Single doses of 10-30 grams of zinc can be fatal.

Special precautions and warnings:

Infants and children: Zinc is **LIKELY SAFE** when taken by mouth appropriately in the recommended amounts. Zinc is **POSSIBLY UNSAFE** when used in high doses.

Pregnancy and breast-feeding: Zinc is **LIKELY SAFE** for most pregnant and breast-feeding women when used in the recommended daily amounts (RDA). However, zinc is **POSSIBLY UNSAFE** when used in high doses by breast-feeding women and **LIKELY UNSAFE** when used in high doses by pregnant women. Pregnant women over 18 should not take more than 40 mg of zinc per day; pregnant women age 14 to 18 should not take more than 34 mg per day. Breast-feeding women over 18 should not take more than 40 mg of zinc per day; breast-feeding women age 14 to 18 should not take more than 34 mg per day.

Alcoholism: Long-term, excessive alcohol drinking is linked to poor zinc absorption in the body.

Diabetes: Large doses of zinc can lower blood sugar in people with diabetes. People with diabetes should use zinc products cautiously.

Haemodialysis: People receiving haemodialysis treatments seem to be at risk for zinc deficiency and might require zinc supplements.

HIV (human immunodeficiency virus) / AIDS: Use zinc cautiously if you have HIV / AIDS. Zinc use has been linked to shorter survival time in people with HIV / AIDs.

Syndromes in which it is difficult for the body to absorb nutrients: People with malabsorption syndromes may be zinc deficient.

Rheumatoid arthritis (RA): People with RA aborb less zinc.

Antibiotics: Quinolone antibiotics interact with zinc, which might decrease how much antibiotic the body absorbs. Taking zinc along with quinalone antibiotics might decrease the effectiveness of these antibiotics. To avoid this interaction take zinc supplements at least 1 hour after antibiotics.

Quinalone antibiotics include ciprofloxacin (Cipro), enoxacin (Penetrex), norfloxacin (Chibroxin, Noroxin), sparfloxacin (Zagam), trovafloxacin (Trovan), and grepafloxacin (Raxar).

Antibiotics: Tetracycline antibiotics interact with zinc, which can attach to tetracyclines in the stomach. This decreases the amount of tetracyclines that can be absorbed. Taking zinc with tetracyclines might decrease the effectiveness of tetracyclines. To avoid this interaction take zinc 2 hours before or 4 hours after taking tetracyclines.

Some tetracyclines include demeclocycline (Declomycin), minocycline (Minocin), and tetracycline (Achromycin).

Cisplatin (Platinol-AQ) interacts with zinc. This agent is used to treat cancer. Taking zinc along with EDTA and cisplatin (Platinol-AQ) might increase the effects and side effects of cisplatin (Platinol-AQ).

Penicillamine interacts with zinc. This agent is used for Wilson's disease and rheumatoid arthritis. Zinc might decrease how much penicillamine your body absorbs and decrease the effectiveness of penicillamine.

Amiloride (Midamor) interacts with zinc. This agent is used as a 'water pill' to help remove excess fluid from the body. Another effect of amiloride is that it can increase the amount of zinc in the body. Taking zinc supplements with amiloride might cause you to have too much zinc in your body.

Magnesium

Magnesium is **LIKELY SAFE** for most people when taken by mouth appropriately or when the prescription-only, injectable product is used correctly. In some people, magnesium might cause stomach upset, nausea, vomiting, diarrhoea, and other side effects.

Doses less than 350 mg per day are safe for most adults. When taken in very large amounts, magnesium is **POSSIBLY UNSAFE**. Large doses might cause too much magnesium to build up in the body, causing serious side effects including an irregular heartbeat, low blood pressure, confusion, slowed breathing, coma, and death.

Special precautions and warnings:

Pregnancy and breast-feeding: Magnesium is **LIKELY SAFE** for pregnant or breast-feeding women when taken by mouth in the recommended amounts. These amounts depend on the age of the woman. Check with your healthcare provider to find out what amounts are right for you.

Bleeding disorders: Magnesium seems to slow blood clotting. In theory, taking magnesium might increase the risk of bleeding or bruising in people with bleeding disorders.

Heart block: High doses of magnesium (typically delivered by IV) should not be given to people with heart block.

Kidney problems, such as kidney failure: Kidneys that don't work well have trouble clearing magnesium from the body. Taking extra magnesium can cause magnesium to build up to dangerous levels. Don't take magnesium if you have kidney problems.

Aminoglycoside antibiotics interact with magnesium, by affecting the muscles. Examples of these antibiotics include amikacin (Amikin), gentamicin (Garamycin), kanamycin (Kantrex), streptomycin, and tobramycin (Nebcin).

Quinolone antibiotics interact with magnesium, which might decrease the amount of antibiotic the body absorbs, thereby reducing the antibiotic's effectiveness. To avoid this interaction take these antibiotics at least 2 hours before, or 4 to 6 hours after, magnesium supplements.

Examples of quinolone antibiotics include ciprofloxacin (Cipro), enoxacin (Penetrex), norfloxacin (Chibroxin, Noroxin), sparfloxacin (Zagam), trovafloxacin (Trovan), and grepafloxacin (Raxar).

Tetracycline antibiotics interact with magnesium, which can attach itself to the antibiotic in the stomach, thus reducing the amount of antibiotic absorbable by the body. To avoid this interaction take magnesium 2 hours before or 4 hours after taking tetracyclines.

Examples of tetracyclines include demeclocycline (Declomycin), minocycline (Minocin), and tetracycline (Achromycin).

Bisphosphonates interact with magnesium, which can reduce the amount of bisphosphate the body absorbs.To avoid this interaction take bisphosphonate at least two hours before magnesium or later in the day.

Examples of bisphosphonates include alendronate (Fosamax), etidronate (Didronel), risedronate (Actonel), tiludronate (Skelid), and others.

Medications for high blood pressure (calcium channel blockers) interact with magnesium, which might decrease blood pressure.

Examples of medications for high blood pressure include nifedipine (Adalat, Procardia), verapamil (Calan, Isoptin, Verelan), diltiazem (Cardizem), isradipine (DynaCirc), felodipine (Plendil), amlodipine (Norvasc), and others.

Muscle relaxants interact with magnesium, which seems to help relax muscles. Taking magnesium along with muscle relaxants can increase the risk of incurring side effects.

Examples of such muscle relaxants include carisoprodol (Soma), pipecuronium (Arduan), orphenadrine (Banflex, Disipal), cyclobenzaprine, gallamine (Flaxedil), atracurium (Tracrium), pancuronium (Pavulon), succinylcholine (Anectine), and others.

Water pills (potassium-sparing diuretics) interact with magnesium. Some water pills can increase the amount of magnesium in the body to unsafe levels.

Examples of such water pills include amiloride (Midamor), spironolactone (Aldactone), and triamterene (Dyrenium).

Vitamin D

Vitamin D is **LIKELY SAFE** when taken by mouth or given as a shot into the muscle in recommended amounts. Most people do not commonly experience side effects with vitamin D, unless too much is taken. Some side effects of taking too much vitamin D include weakness, fatigue, sleepiness, headache, loss of appetite, dry mouth, metallic taste, nausea, vomiting, and others.

Taking vitamin D for long periods of time in doses higher than 4000 units daily is **POSSIBLY UNSAFE** and may cause excessively high levels of calcium in the blood. However, much higher doses are often needed for the short-term treatment of vitamin D deficiency. This type of treatment should be done under the supervision of a healthcare provider.

Special precautions and warnings:

Pregnancy and breast-feeding. Vitamin D is **LIKELY SAFE** during pregnancy and breast-feeding when used in daily amounts below 4000 units. Do not use higher doses. Vitamin D is **POSSIBLY UNSAFE** when used in higher amounts during pregnancy or while breast-feeding. Using higher doses might cause serious harm to the infant.

Kidney disease. Vitamin D may increase calcium levels and increase the risk of 'hardening of the arteries' in people with serious kidney disease. This must be balanced with the need to prevent renal osteodystrophy, a bone disease that occurs when the kidneys fail to maintain the proper levels of calcium and phosphorus in the blood. Levels of calcium in people with kidney disease should be monitored carefully.

High levels of calcium in the blood. Taking vitamin D could make this condition worse.

'Hardening of the arteries' (atherosclerosis). Taking vitamin D could make this condition worse, especially in people with kidney disease.

Sarcoidosis. Vitamin D may increase calcium levels in people with sarcoidosis. This could lead to kidney stones and other problems. Use vitamin D cautiously.

Histoplasmosis: Vitamin D may increase calcium levels in people with histoplasmosis. This could lead to kidney stones and other problems. Use vitamin D cautiously.

Over-active parathyroid gland (hyperparathyroidism). Vitamin D may increase calcium levels in people with hyperparathyroidism. Use vitamin D cautiously.

Lymphoma. Vitamin D may increase calcium levels in people with lymphoma. This could lead to kidney stones and other problems. Use vitamin D cautiously.

Tuberculosis. Vitamin D might increase calcium levels in people with tuberculosis. This might result in complications such as kidney stones.

Minor interactions

Cimetidine (Tagamet) interacts with Vitamin D; it may decrease how well the body converts Vitamin D into useable agents. However, for most people this is probably not significant.

Heparin interacts with Vitamin D. This agent slows blood clotting and can increase the risk of breaking a bone when used for a long period of time. People taking this medication should eat a diet rich in calcium and vitamin D.

Low molecular weight heparins (LMWHs) interact with Vitamin D. These medications can increase the risk of breaking a bone when used for a long periods of time. People taking these medications should eat a diet rich in calcium and vitamin D.

Examples of these drugs include enoxaparin (Lovenox), dalteparin (Fragmin), and tinzaparin (Innohep).

Calcium

Calcium is **LIKELY SAFE** for most people when taken by mouth or when given intravenously and appropriately. It can cause some minor side effects such as belching or gas.

Calcium is **POSSIBLY UNSAFE** for both children and adults when taken by mouth in high doses. Avoid taking too much calcium. The Institute of Medicine sets the daily tolerable upper intake level (UL) for calcium based on age as follows: Age 0-6 months, 1000 mg; 6-12 months, 1500 mg;

1-3 years, 2500 mg; 9-18 years, 3000 mg; 19-50 years, 2500 mg; 51+ years, 2000 mg. Higher doses increase the chance of having serious side effects. Some recent research also suggests that doses over the recommended daily requirement of 1000-1300 mg daily for most adults might increase the chance of heart attack. This research does suggest cause for concern, but it is still too soon to say for certain that calcium is truly the cause of heart attack. Until more is known, continue consuming adequate amounts of calcium to meet daily requirements, but not excessive amounts of calcium. Be sure to consider total calcium intake from both dietary and supplemental sources and try not to exceed 1000-1300 mg of calcium per day. To figure out dietary calcium, count 300 mg / day from non-dairy foods plus 300 mg / cup of milk or fortified orange juice.

Special precautions and warnings:

Pregnancy and breast-feeding Calcium is **LIKELY SAFE** when taken by mouth in recommended amounts during pregnancy and breast-feeding. There is not enough information available on the safety of using calcium intravenously (by IV) during pregnancy and breastfeeding.

Low acid levels in the stomach (achlorhydria). People with low levels of gastric acid absorb less calcium if calcium is taken on an empty stomach. However, low acid levels in the stomach do not appear to reduce calcium absorption if calcium is taken with food. Advise people with achlorhydria to take calcium supplements with meals.

High levels of phosphate in the blood (hyperphosphatemia) or low levels of phosphate in the blood (hypophosphatemia). Calcium and phosphate have to be in balance in the body. Taking too much calcium can throw this balance off and cause harm. Don't take extra calcium without your health provider's supervision.

Poor kidney function. Calcium supplementation can increase the risk of having too much calcium in the blood in people with poor kidney function.

Too much calcium in the blood (as in parathyroid gland disorders and sarcoidosis). Calcium should be avoided if you have one of these conditions.

Smoking. People who smoke absorb less calcium from the stomach.

Under-active thyroid (hypothyroidism). Calcium can interfere with thyroid hormone replacement treatment. Separate calcium and thyroid medications by at least 4 hours.

Major Interaction

Ceftriaxone (Rocephin) interacts with calcium. Administering intravenous ceftriaxone and calcium can result in life-threatening damage to the lungs and kidneys. Calcium should not be administered intravenously within 48 hours of intravenous ceftriaxone.

Moderate Interaction

Quinolone antibiotics interact with calcium, which might decrease how much antibiotic your body absorbs and thereby reduce antibiotic effectiveness. To avoid this interaction, take calcium supplements at least one hour after antibiotics.

Examples of quinolone antibiotics include ciprofloxacin (Cipro), enoxacin (Penetrex), norfloxacin (Chibroxin, Noroxin), sparfloxacin (Zagam), and trovafloxacin (Trovan).

Tetracycline antibiotics interact with calcium, which can attach to tetracycline in the stomach, reducing its effectiveness. To avoid this interaction take calcium 2 hours before or 4 hours after taking tetracyclines.

Examples of tetracyclines include demeclocycline (Declomycin), minocycline (Minocin), and tetracycline (Achromycin, and others).

Bisphosphonates interact with calcium, which can reduce the amount of bisphosphate your body absorbs. Taking calcium along with bisphosphates can decrease the effectiveness of bisphosphate. To avoid this interaction, take bisphosphonate at least 30 minutes before calcium or later in the day.

Some bisphosphonates include alendronate (Fosamax), etidronate (Didronel), risedronate (Actonel), tiludronate (Skelid), and others.

Calcipotriene (Dovonex) interacts with calcium. Just like vitamin D, calcipotriene helps your body absorb calcium. Taking calcium supplements along with calcipotriene might cause the body to have too much calcium.

Digoxin (Lanoxin) interacts with calcium. Calcium can affect your heart. Digoxin is used to help your heart beat stronger. Taking calcium along with digoxin might increase the effects of digoxin and lead to an irregular heartbeat. If you are taking digoxin, talk to your doctor before taking calcium supplements.

Diltiazem (Cardizem, Dilacor, Tiazac) interacts with calcium. Both calcium and diltiazem can affect the heart. Taking large amounts of calcium along with diltiazem might decrease the effectiveness of diltiazem.

Levothyroxine interacts with calcium. Levothyroxine is used for low thyroid function. Calcium can decrease how much levothyroxine your body absorbs. Taking calcium along with levothyroxine might decrease the effectiveness of levothyroxine. Levothyroxine and calcium should be taken at least 4 hours apart.

Some brands that contain levothyroxine include Armour Thyroid, Eltroxin, Estre, Euthyrox, Levo-T, Levothroid, Levoxyl, Synthroid, Unithroid, and others.

Sotalol (Betapace) interacts with calcium. Taking calcium with sotalol can decrease how much sotalol your body absorbs, or decrease the effectiveness of sotalol. To avoid this inter-action, take calcium at least 2 hours before or 4 hours after taking sotalol.

Verapamil (Calan, Covera, Isoptin, Verelan) interacts with calcium. Calcium can affect your heart. Verapamil can also affect your heart. Do not take large amounts of calcium if you are taking verapamil.

Water pills (Thiazide diuretics) interact with calcium. Some 'water pills' increase the amount of calcium in your body. Taking large amounts of calcium with some water pills might cause there to be too much calcium in the body. resulting in serious side effects, including kidney problems.

Examples of these water pills include chlorothiazide (Diuril), hydrochlorothiazide (HydroDIURIL, Esidrix), indapamide (Lozol), metolazone (Zaroxolyn), and chlorthalidone (Hygroton).

Minor Interaction

Oestrogens interact with calcium. Oestrogen helps your body absorb calcium. Taking oestrogen pills along with large amounts of calcium might increase calcium in the body too much.

Oestrogen pills include conjugated equine oestrogens (Premarin), ethinyl estradiol, estradiol, and others.

Medications for high blood pressure (calcium channel blockers) interact with calcium. Some medications for high blood pressure, known as calcium channel blockers, affect calcium in your body. Getting calcium injections might decrease the effectiveness of these medications.

Some medications for high blood pressure include nifedipine (Adalat, Procardia), verapamil (Calan, Isoptin, Verelan), diltiazem (Cardizem), isradipine (DynaCirc), felodipine (Plendil), amlodipine (Norvasc), and others.

5-HTP

5-HTP is **POSSIBLY SAFE** when taken by mouth. However, some people who have taken it have come down with eosinophilia-myalgia syndrome (EMS), a serious condition involving extreme muscle tenderness (myalgia) and blood abnormalities (eosinophilia). Some people think EMS might be caused by an accidental ingredient (contaminant) in some 5-HTP products. However, there is not enough scientific evidence to know if EMS is caused by 5-HTP, a contaminant, or some other factor. Until more is known, 5-HTP should be used cautiously.

Other potential side effects of 5-HTP include heartburn, stomach pain, nausea, vomiting, diarrhoea, drowsiness, sexual problems, and muscle problems.

Special precautions and warnings:

Pregnancy and breast-feeding: 5-HTP is **POSSIBLY UNSAFE** when taken by mouth when pregnant or breast-feeding. Avoid using it in these circumstances.

Down's syndrome: There are reports of 5-HTP causing seizures in some people with Down's syndrome. In one group studied, 15% of people with Down's syndrome receiving long-term 5-HTP treatment experienced seizures.

Surgery: 5-HTP can affect the brain chemical serotonin,

which can also be affected by some drugs administered during surgery. Taking 5-HTP before surgery might cause too much serotonin in the brain and can result in serious side effects including heart problems, shivering, and anxiety. Patients should stop taking 5-HTP at least 2 weeks before surgery.

Major interaction

Medications for depression (antidepressant drugs) interact with 5-HTP. 5-HTP increases a brain chemical called serotonin, which is also increased by some medications for depression. Taking 5-HTP along with these antidepressant drugs might increase serotonin too much and cause serious side effects including heart problems, shivering and anxiety. Do not take 5-HTP if you are taking antidepressant drugs.

Examples of these medications for depression include fluoxetine (Prozac), paroxetine (Paxil), sertraline (Zoloft), amitriptyline (Elavil), clomipramine (Anafranil), imipramine (Tofranil), and others.

Medications for depression (monoamine oxidase inhibitors, or MAOIs) interact with 5-HTP. 5-HTP increases the brain chemical serotonin, as do MAOIs. Taking 5-HTP with these medications might cause there to be too much serotonin. This could cause serious side effects including heart problems, shivering, and anxiety.

Examples of MAOIs include phenelzine (Nardil), tranylcypromine (Parnate), and others.

Moderate interaction

Carbidopa (Lodosyn) interacts with 5-HTP. Both 5-HTP and cardidopa can affect the brain. Taking 5-HTP along with carbidopa can increase the risk of serious side effects including rapid speech, anxiety, aggressiveness, and others.

Dextromethorphan (Robitussin DM, and others) interacts with 5-HTP. 5-HTP can affect the brain chemical serotonin, as does dextromethorphan. Taking 5-HTP along with dextromethorphan might cause too much serotonin in the brain and serious side effects including heart problems, shivering and anxiety. Do not take 5-HTP if you are taking dextromethorphan.

Meperidine (Demerol) interacts with 5-HTP. Both 5-HTP and meperidine increase the brain chemical serotonin. Taking 5-HTP along with meperidine might cause there to be too much serotonin in the brain, resulting in serious side effects including heart problems, shivering, and anxiety.

Pentazocine (Talwin) interacts with 5-HTP. Both 5-HTP and pentazocine increase the brain chemical serotonin. Taking both together might increase serotonin too much, which could cause serious side effects including heart problems, shivering, and anxiety. Do not take 5-HTP if you are taking pentazocine.

Tramadol (Ultram) interacts with 5-HTP. Both tramadol and 5-HTP affect the brain chemical serotonin. Taking 5-HTP along with tramadol might cause too much serotonin in the brain and side effects including confusion, shivering, stiff muscles, and others.

Fish Oil/ DHA

Fish oil is **LIKELY SAFE** for most people, including pregnant and breast-feeding women, when taken in low doses (3 grams or less per day). There are some safety concerns when fish oil is taken in high doses. Taking more than 3 grams per day might keep blood from clotting and can increase the chance of bleeding.

High doses of fish oil might also reduce the immune

system's activity, reducing the body's ability to fight infection. This is a special concern for people taking medications to reduce their immune system's activity (organ transplant patients, for example) and the elderly.

Only take high doses of fish oil while under medical supervision.

Fish oil can cause side effects including belching, bad breath, heartburn, nausea, loose stools, rash, and nose-bleeds. Taking fish oil supplements with meals or freezing them can often decrease these side effects.

Consuming large amounts of fish oil from some dietary sources is **POSSIBLY UNSAFE**. Some fish meats (especially shark, king mackerel, and farm-raised salmon) can be contaminated with mercury and other industrial and environ-mental chemicals, but fish oil supplements typically do not contain these contaminants.

Special precautions and warnings:

Liver disease: Fish oil might increase the risk of bleeding in people with liver scarring due to liver disease.

Fish or seafood allergy: Some people who are allergic to seafood such as fish might also be allergic to fish oil sup-plements. There is no reliable information showing how likely people with seafood allergy are to have an allergic reaction to fish oil. Until more is known, advise patients allergic to seafood to avoid or use fish oil supplements cautiously.

Bipolar disorder: Taking fish oil might increase some of the symptoms of this condition.

Depression: Taking fish oil might increase some of the symptoms of this condition.

Diabetes: There is some concern that taking high doses of fish oil might make the control of blood sugar more difficult.

High blood pressure: Fish oil can lower blood pressure and might cause blood pressure to drop too low in people who are being treated with blood pressure-lowering medications.

HIV / AIDS and other conditions in which the immune system response is lowered: Higher doses of fish oil can lower the body's immune system response. This could be a problem for people whose immune system is already weak.

An implanted defibrillator (a surgically placed device to prevent irregular heartbeat): some, but not all, research suggests that fish oil might increase the risk of irregular heartbeat in patients with an implanted defibrillator. Stay on the safe side by avoiding fish oil supplements.

Familial adenomatous polyposis: There is some concern that fish oil might further increase the risk of getting cancer in people with this condition.

Moderate Interaction

Birth control pills (contraceptive drugs) interact with fish oil. Fish oils seem to help reduce some fat levels in the blood. These fats are called triglycerides. Birth control pills might decrease the effectiveness of fish oils by reducing these fat levels in the blood.

Examples of birth control pills include ethinyl estradiol & levonorgestrel (Triphasil), ethinyl estradiol & norethindrone (Ortho-Novum 1/35, Ortho-Novum 7/7/7), and others.

Medications for high blood pressure (antihypertensive drugs) interact with fish oil. Fish oils seem to decrease blood pressure. Taking fish oils along with medications for high blood pressure might cause your blood pressure to go too low.

Examples of medications for high blood pressure include captopril (Capoten), enalapril (Vasotec), losartan (Cozaar), valsartan (Diovan), diltiazem (Cardizem), Amlodipine (Norvasc), hydrochlorothiazide (HydroDiuril), furosemide (Lasix), and many others.

Orlistat (Xenical, Alli) interacts with fish oil. Orlistat is used for weight loss. It prevents dietary fats from being absorbed from the gut. There is some concern that orlistat might also decrease absorption of fish oil when they are taken together. To avoid this potential interaction take orlistat and fish oil at least 2 hours apart.

Mild Interaction

Medications that slow blood clotting (anticoagulant / antiplatelet drugs) interact with fish oil. Fish oils might slow blood clotting. Taking fish oils along with medications that also slow clotting might increase the chances of bruising and bleeding.

Examples of medications that slow blood clotting include aspirin, clopidogrel (Plavix), diclofenac (Voltaren, Cataflam, others), ibuprofen (Advil, Motrin, others), naproxen (Anaprox, Naprosyn, others), dalteparin (Fragmin), heparin, enoxaparin (Lovenox), warfarin (Coumadin), and others.

CLA

Conjugated linoleic acid is **LIKELY SAFE** when taken by mouth in amounts found in foods and is **POSSIBLY SAFE** when taken by mouth in medicinal amounts (larger amounts than those found in food). It might cause side effects such as stomach upset, diarrhoea, nausea, and fatigue.

Special precautions and warnings:

Children. Conjugated linoleic acid is **POSSIBLY SAFE** for children when taken by mouth in medicinal amounts for up to 7 months. There is not enough evidence to know if long-term use is safe.

Pregnancy and breast-feeding. Conjugated linoleic acid is **LIKELY SAFE** when taken by mouth in food amounts. But there is not enough evidence to know if conjugated linoleic acid is safe to use in medicinal mounts during pregnancy and breast-feeding. Stay on the safe side and avoid use.

Bleeding disorders. Conjugated linoleic acid might slow blood clotting. In theory, conjugated linoleic acid might increase the risk of bruising and bleeding in people with bleeding disorders.

Diabetes. There are concerns that taking conjugated linoleic acid can worsen diabetes. Avoid use if diabetic.

Metabolic syndrome. There are concerns that taking conjugated linoleic acid might increase the risk of getting diabetes if you have metabolic syndrome. Avoid use.

Surgery. Conjugated linoleic acid might cause extra bleeding during and after surgery. Stop using it at least two weeks before a scheduled surgery.

Nitro+ Diet Medical & Exercise Disclaimer

1. No advice

The Nitro+ Diet contains general information about medical conditions, nutrition, exercises, health and diets. The information is not advice and should not be treated as such.

2. No warranties

The medical information in the Nitro+ Diet is provided without any representations or warranties, express or implied. We make no representations or warranties in relation to the medical information in this book.

We do not warrant or represent that the medical information in this book is complete, true, accurate, up to date and / or non-misleading.

3. Professional assistance

Before starting the Nitro+ Diet and exercise programme we strongly recommend you speak to your doctor or physician – especially if you answer yes to any of the questions below.

- Do you feel pain in your chest when you do physical activity?
- Have you been told by your doctor that you should only do physical activity recommended by a doctor because you have a heart condition?
- Have you had any chest pain in the past month when not doing physical activity?
- Do you lose your balance as a result of dizziness or do you ever lose consciousness/collapse?
- Do you have a bone or joint problem (e.g. back, knee, or hip) that could be made worse by exercise?
- Is your doctor currently prescribing medication for your blood pressure or heart condition?

- Do you know of any other reason why you should not do physical activity?

You should never delay seeking medical advice, disregard medical advice or discontinue medical treatment because of information in this book.

4. Limiting our liability

Nothing in this medical & exercise disclaimer will:

a) limit any of our liabilities in any way that is not permitted under applicable law; or

b) exclude any of our liabilities that may not be excluded under applicable law.

You must not rely on the information outlined in this book as an alternative to medical advice from your doctor or other professional healthcare provider. If you have any specific questions about any medical matter, you should consult your doctor or other professional healthcare provider. Please also discuss with your doctor the supplements that are suggested and confirm that you can safely take these in the dosages specified. If you are not sure about any of the supplements you will find all contraindications for each supplement in Appendix C.

If you think you may be suffering from any medical condition, you should seek immediate medical attention.

The diet is not recommended for the following:

- People who are underweight or have an eating disorder.
- Children (under 18 years old).
- Type 1 diabetics and diabetics taking medication for their diabetes (other than Metformin).

- Pregnant women or breast-feeding mothers.
- People recovering from surgery.
- Those who are frail or have a significant underlying medical condition should speak to their doctor first, as they would before embarking on any weight-loss regime.
- Those who are not sure about whether it may affect their prescribed medications should to speak to their doctor first.
- People feeling unwell or have a fever.
- Those taking Warfarin should consult their doctor first as it may increase their INR.

Sources & References

Nitrogen foods

Ensselaer Polytechnic Institute: *Amino Acid Catabolism: Nitrogen*

Allegheny University of Health Sciences: *Purine and Pyrimidine Metabolism*

MedlinePlus: *Protein in Diet*

Drugs.com: *Low Purine Diet*

Colorado State Extension: *Omega-3 Fatty Acids*

American Journal of Clinical Nutrition: *Meta-Analysis of Nitrogen Balance Studies for Estimating Protein Requirements in Healthy Adults*

Nitrogen balance

Weinheimer E. M., Sands L. P., Campbell W. W. (2010) *A systematic review of the separate and combined effects of energy restriction and exercise on fat-free mass in middle-aged and older adults: implications for sarcopenic obesity.* Nutr. Rev. 68, 375–388

Ebbeling C. B., Swain J. F., Feldman H. A., Wong W. W., Hachey D. L., Garcia-Lago E.,Ludwig D. S.: *Effects of dietary composition on energy expenditure during weight-loss maintenance.* JAMA 2012, 307, 2627–2634

Ravussin E., Lillioja S., Knowler W. C., Christin L., Freymond D., Abbott W. G.,Boyce V., Howard B. V., Bogardus C.: *Reduced rate of energy expenditure as a risk factor for body-weight gain.* N. Engl. J. Med. 1988, 318, 467–472

Stein T. P., Rumpler W. V., Leskiw M. J., Schluter M. D., Staples R., Bodwell C. E.: *Effect of reduced dietary intake on energy expenditure, protein turnover, and glucose cycling in man.* Metabolism 1991, 40, 478–483

Protein RDAs

Hermann, Janice R. *Protein and the Body* Oklahoma Cooperative Extension Service, Division of Agricultural Sciences and Natural Resources, Oklahoma State University: T–3163–1 – T–3163–4.

Food and Nutrition Board. *A Report of the Panel on Macronutrients, Subcommittees on Upper Reference Levels of Nutrients and Interpretation and Uses of Dietary Reference Intakes, and the Standing Committee on the Scientific Evaluation of Dietary Reference Intakes.* The National Academies Press, Washington D.C. (2005)

Nutrition Working Group of the International Olympic Committee IOC Consensus Conference on Nutrition for Sport, Lausanne (2003)

Global obesity crisis

World Health Organization: *Global Health Observatory Data repository*

UK Department of Health, 2014: *Obesity and Healthy Eating*

Analysis of overweight and obesity data, Institute for Health Metrics and Evaluation (IHME) at the University of Washington.

Diet and obesity

NHS Information Booklet: *Statistics on Obesity, Physical Activity and Diet.* UK, 2006.

www.ic.nhs.uk/webfiles/publications/opan06/OPAN%20bulletin%20finalv2.pdf

Ludwig DS et al: *Relation Between Consumption of Sugar-sweetened Drinks and Childhood Obesity: a prospective, observational analysis.* Lancet 2001; 357, 505-508

James J et al: *Preventing Childhood Obesity by Reducing Consumption of Carbonated Drinks: Cluster Randomised Controlled Trial.* British Medical Journal 2004; 328,1237

Karppanen H, Mervaala E: *Sodium Intake and Hypertension.* Prog Cardiovasc Dis. 2006; 49, 59-75

Obesity and the NHS

National Audit Office: *Tackling Obesity in England.* The Stationery

Office, London, 2001

Butland B, Jebb S, Kopelman P, et al: *Tackling obesities: future choices – project report (2nd Ed)*. Foresight Programme of the Government Office for Science, London, 2007

Weighing up the burden of obesity: a review. Dr Foster Research, London, 2008

Preventing overweight and obesity in Scotland: a route map towards healthy weight. The Scottish Government, Edinburgh, 2010

House of Commons Health Committee: *Obesity: Third Report of Session 2003/4.* The Stationery Office, London, 2004

Morgan, E and Dent, M: *The economic burden of obesity.* National Obesity Observatory, Oxford, 2010

Obesity and heart disease

Estes EH Jr, Seider HO, McIntosh HD: *Reversible cardiopulmonary syndrome with extreme obesity.* Circulation, 1957;16:179-187.

Matts JP, Buchwald H, Fitch LL, Campos CT, Varco RL, Campbell GS, Pearce MB, YellinAE, Smink RD Jr, Sawin HS Jr, Long JM. *Subgroup analyses of the major clinical endpoints in the program on the surgical control of the hyperlipidemias (Posch): overall mortality, atherosclerotic coronary heart disease (ACHD) mortality, and ACHD mortality or myocardial infarction.* J Clin Epidemiol 1995; 48:389-405.

Acid reflux / Gerd

Jacobson, B. New England Journal of Medicine, June 1, 2006; vol 354: pp 2340-2348.

Kaltenbach, T. Archives of Internal Medicine, May 8, 2006; vol 166: pp 965-971.

Hampel, H. Annals of Internal Medicine, Aug. 2, 2005; vol 143: pp 199-211.

Murray, L. International Journal of Epidemiology, August 2003; vol 32: pp 645-650.

Sacks, F. New England Journal of Medicine, Feb. 26, 2009; vol 360: pp 859-873.

Cancer

www.cancerresearchuk.org

Leptin resistance

Richard Atkinson, MD, clinical professor of pathology, Virginia Commonwealth University.

Robert H. Lustig, MD, professor of pediatrics, University of California, San Francisco; member, Endocrine Society's Obesity Task Force.

Ellerhorst, J. *Oncology Reports*, April 2010: pp. 901-907.

http://www.webmd.com/diet/the-facts-on-leptin-faq?page=1

Preparing the system

Angulo P. *GI epidemiology: nonalcoholic fatty liver disease.* Aliment Pharmacol Ther. 2007;25(8):883-9. doi:10.1111/j.1365-2036.-2007.03246.x

Anstee QM, Targher G, Day CP. *Progression of NAFLD to diabetes mellitus, cardiovascular disease or cirrhosis.* Nat Rev Gastroenterol Hepatol.

Sargent S. *Liver diseases: an essential guide for nurses and health care professionals.* 2009:1-359.

Takei Y. *Treatment of non-alcoholic fatty liver disease.* J Gastroenterol Hepatol. 2013;28 Suppl 4:79-80. doi:10.1111/jgh.12242.

Lean Body Mass calculation

Hume, R *Prediction of lean body mass from height and weight.* Journal of clinical pathology 19 (Jul 1966): 389-91.

Fuchs, RJ; Theis, CF; Lancaster, MC. *A nomogram to predict lean body mass in men.* The American journal of clinical nutrition 31-4 (Apr 1978): 673–8.

Skin Fold Measurements

Jackson, A.S. & Pollock, M.L. *Generalized equations for predicting body density of men.* British J of Nutrition, 40 (1978): p497-504.

Jackson, et al. *Generalized equations for predicting body density of women.* Medicine and Science in Sports and Exercise 12 (1980): p175-182.

Why the PNB diet is safe

Bilsborough S1, Mann N. *Review of issues of dietary protein intake in humans.* Int J Sport Nutr Exerc Metab. 2006 Apr;16(2):129-52.A

Diabetes

WEB MD- Diabetes Health Center

Hypertension and Cardiovascular Disease

Swithers SE, Patterson NA. *Artificial sweeteners produce the counter-intuitive effect of inducing metabolic derangements.* Trends in Endocrinology & Metabolism 2013.

Vegetable digestibility

Dietary Reference Intakes for Energy, Carbohydrate, Fiber, Fat, Fatty Acids, Cholesterol, Protein, and Amino Acids, Food and Drug Administration, Institute of Medicine of the National Academies, 2005.

Fat & Energy

Colgan, Dr Michael: *Optimum sports nutrition- battling the bulge.* Advanced Research Pi, 1993

http://www.ncbi.nlm.nih.gov/pmc/articles/PMC3257631/

Tucker L.A., Thomas K.S. *Increasing total fiber intake reduces risk of weight and fat gains in women.* J. Nutr. 2009;139:576–58

Liu R.H. *Health benefits of fruit and vegetables are from additive and synergistic combinations of phytochemicals.* Am. J. Clin. Nutr. 2003; 78:517S–520

Ogden C.L., Carroll M.D., Curtin L.R., McDowell M.A., Tabak C.J., Flegal K.M. *Prevalence of overweight and obesity in the United States, 1999–2004.* J. Am. Med. Assoc. 2006; 295:1549–1555

Li Z., Bowerman S., Heber D. *Health ramifications of the obesity epidemic.* Surg. Clin. North Am. 2005; 85:681–701.

Ahlborg B, et al. *Muscle glycogen and electrolytes during prolonged physical exercise,* Acta PhysiolScand 1967; 70:129-142

Protein

Holford, Patrick: *The New Optimum Nutrition Bible* Crossing Press; rev edition 2005

Dangin M, Boirie Y, Garcia-Rodenas C, Gachon P, Fauquant J, Callier P, Ballevre O, Beaufrere B. *The digestion rate of protein is an independent regulating factor of postprandial protein retention.* Am J Physiol Endocrinol Metab 280-2 (2001): E340-8.

Boirie Y, Dangin M, Gachon P, Vasson MP, Maubois JL, Beaufrere B. *Slow and fast dietary proteins differently modulate postprandial protein accretion.* Proc Natl Acad Sci USA. 1997, 94(26):14930-5.

Willoughby DS, Stout JR, Wilborn CD. *Effects of resistance training and protein plus amino acid supplementation on muscle anabolism, mass, and strength.* Amino Acids. 2006 Sep 20.

Bilsborough S1, Mann N. *A Review of Issues of Dietary Protein Intake in Humans* Int J Sport Nutr Exerc Metab. 16-2 (2006): 129-52

www.consumerreports.org/cro/2012/04/protein-drinks/

Leidy HJ, Hoertel HA, Douglas SM, Shafer RS. *Daily addition of a protein-rich breakfast for long-term improvements in energy intake regulation and body weight management in overweight & obese 'breakfast skipping' young people.* Experimental Biology, Boston, MA. April 20 2013

Karalus, M, et al. *The effect of commercially prepared breakfast meals with varying levels of protein on acute satiety in non-restrained women.* Abstract presented at Experimental Biology, 2014.

Leidy H, et al. *Acute Effects of High Protein, Sausage and Egg-based Convenience Breakfast Meals on Postprandial Glucose Homeostasis in Healthy, Premenopausal Women.* Abstract presented at Experimental Biology, 2014.

Zinc

Biol Trace Elem Res. 2013 Aug;154(2):168-77

Chromium Picolinate

Mertz W, SHpcott D, Hubert J, eds. *Chromium in Nutrition and*

Metabolism. Amsterdam: Elseviar N.Hollan 1979:11.

Press RI, Geller J, Evans GW. *The effect of chromium picolinate on serum cholesterol and apolipoprotein fractions in human subjects.* Western J Med 1990; 152:41-45

Colgan, Michael: *Optimum Sport Nutrition, Chromium Picolinate has Anabolic Effects (page 318)* Advanced Research Press Inc., U.S. 1993

5-HTP

Cangiano C, Ceci F, Cairella M, Cascino A, Del Ben M, Laviano A, Muscaritoli M, Rossi-Fanelli F. *Effects of 5-hydroxytryptophan on eating behavior and adherence to dietary prescriptions in obese adult subjects.* Adv Exp Med Biol 1991;294:591-3

L-Carnitine

Odo, S., Tanabe, K. & Yamauchi, M. *A Pilot Clinical Trial on L-Carnitine Supplementation in Combination with Motivation Training: Effects on Weight Management in Healthy Volunteers,* Food and Nutrition, Volume 4 (pp. 222-231), 2013

Wutzke, K.D. & Lorenz, H. *The Effect of L-Carnitine on Fat Oxidation, Protein Turnover, and Body Composition in Slightly Overweight Subjects*, Metabolism, Vol. 53-8, 2004: pp. 1002-1006

Reda, E., D'Iddio, S., Nicolai, R., Benatti, P. & Calvani, M. *The Carnitine System and Body Composition*, Acta Diabetol 40, 2003: pp. 106-113

Earle, RW, & Baechle, TR (eds), *NSCAs Essentials of Personal Training*, NSCA, 2004

Caffeine

Lee, J.B., Bae, J.S., Matsumoto, T., Yang, H.M., Min, Y.K. (2009) *Tropical Malaysians and temperate Koreans exhibit significant differences in sweating sensitivity to iontophoretically administered acetylcholine.* Int. J. Biometeorol. 53: pp. 149-157

Horowitz, M. *Heat acclimation: A continuum of process.* In: Mercer, J. ed. *Thermal Physiology.* Elsevier, Amsterdam, 1989: pp. 445-450

Sato, K., Sato, F. *Pharmacologic responsiveness of isolated single eccrine sweat glands.* Am. J. Physiol. 240 (1981): pp. R44-R51

Torres, N.E., Zollman, P.J., Low, P.A. *Characterization of muscarinic receptor subtype of rat eccrine sweat gland by autoradiography.* Brain Res. 550 (1991): pp. 129-132

Nicholson, S.A. *Stimulatory effect of caffeine on the hypothalamopituitary-adrenocortical axis in the rat.* J. Endocrinol. 122 (1989): pp. 535-543

Soeren, M., Mohr, T., Kjaer, M., Graham, T.E. *Acute effects of caffeine ingestion at rest in humans with impaired epinephrine responses.* J. Appl. Physiol. 80 (1996): pp. 999-1005

Weight gain from diet drinks

Fowler SP, Williams K, Resendez RG, Hunt KJ, Hazuda HP, Stern MP. *Fueling the obesity epidemic? Artificially sweetened beverage use and long-term weight gain.* Obesity (Silver Spring) 16-8 (2008): pp 1894-900.

Conjugated Linoleic Acid

Blankson H, Stakkestad JA, Fagertun H, Thom E, Wadstein J, Gudmundsen O: *Conjugated linoleic acid reduces body fat mass in overweight and obese humans.* J Nutr. 130-12 (2000): pp 2943-8.

Glutamine

Prada, P.O., Hirabara, S.M., de Souza, C.T., Schenka, A.A., Zecchin,H.G., Vassallo, J., Velloso, L.A., Carneiro, E., Carvalheira, J.B., Curi, R. & Saad, M.J. *L-glutamine supplementation induces insulin resistance in adipose tissue and improves insulin signalling in liver and muscle with diet-induced obesity,* Diabetologia, Volume 50, issue 9 (2007) pp. 149-159

Bowtell, J.L., Gelly, K., Jackman, M.L., Patel, A., Simeoni, M, Rennie, M.J. *Effect of oral glutamine on whole body carbohydrate storage during recovery from exhaustive exercise,* Journal Of Applied Physiology, Volume 86-6 (1999) pp. 1770-1777

Casein

Astrup, A. et al. *Effect of Short-Term High Dietary Calcium Intake on 24-h Energy Expenditure, Fat Oxidation, and Fecal Fat Excretion.* International Journal of Obesity 29 (2005), pp 292-301.

Demling, R. & DeSanti, L. *Effect of a Hypocaloric Diet, Increased Protein Intake and Resistance Training on Lean Mass Gains and Fat Mass Loss in Overweight Police Officers.* Annals of Nutrition & Metabolism (2000). 44:21-29

Le Leu, R. et al. *Whey Proteins as Functional Food Ingredients.* International Dairy Journal. Vol 0 (1990), Issue 5-6. 425-434

Deutz, N. et al. *Casein and soy protein meals differentially affect whole-body and splanchnic protein metabolism in healthy humans* Journal of Nutrition. Vol. 135-5. 5 (2005) , pp. 1080-1087

Calcium

Heaney RP. *Normalizing calcium intake: projected population effects for body weight.* J Nutr 2003; 133: 268S-270S

Melanson EL, Sharp TA, Schneider J, Donahoo WT, Grunwald GK, Hill JO. *Relation between calcium intake and fat oxidation in adult humans.* Int J Obes Relat Metab Disord 27 (2003): pp 196-203

Papakonstantinou E, Flatt WP, Huth PJ, Harris RBS. *High dietary calcium reduces body fat content, digestibility of fat, and serum* ꟷꟷꟷꟷꟷꟷꟷꟷ ꟷꟷ ꟷꟷ ꟷꟷꟷꟷ ꟷꟷꟷꟷ ꟷꟷꟷ ꟷ ꟷ (ꟷꟷꟷꟷ) ꟷꟷꟷ ꟷꟷ ꟷ ꟷꟷꟷ

Shapses SA, Heshka S, Heymsfield SB. *Effect of calcium supplementation on weight and fat loss in women.* J Clin Endocrinol Metab. 89-2 (2004): pp 632-7

Zemel MB, Thompson W, Milstead A, Morris K, Campbell P. *Calcium and dairy acceleration of weight and fat loss during energy restriction in obese adults.* Obes Res. 12-4 (2004): pp 582-90

Magnesium

Maier JA, Malpuech-Brugere C, Zimowska W, Rayssiguier Y, Mazur A. *Low magnesium promotes endothelial cell dysfunction: implications for atherosclerosis, inflammation and thrombosis.* Biochim Biophys Acta. 24-5 (2004) 1689(1):13-21

Consequences of magnesium deficiency on the enhancement of stress reactions; preventive and therapeutic implications (a review). J Am Coll Nutr. Oct 1994: pp 429-46.

Kinetic Exercise Plan

https://www.acefitness.org/acefit/healthy-living-article/ 60/3543/ why-you-should-be-foam-rolling/

Sullivan KM1, Silvey DB, Button DC, Behm DG. *Roller-massager application to the hamstrings increases sit-and-reach range of motion within five to ten seconds without performance impairments.* Int J Sports Phys Ther. 2013 Jun;8(3): 228-36

Bellew JW, Fenter PC, Chelette B, Moore R, Loreno D. *Effects of a short-term dynamic balance training program in healthy older women.* J Geriatr Phys Ther. 2005; 28(1): 4-8, 27

Hydration

Batmanghelidj, Fereydoon. *Your Body's Many Cries for Water.* Global Health Solutions, 1995

Sleep

Copinschi, G. *Metabolic and endocrine effects of sleep deprivation.* Essent Psychopharmacol. 6-6 (2005): 341-7

Leproult, R., & Van Cauter, E. *Role of Sleep and Sleep Loss In Hormonal Release and Metabolism.* Endocrine Development. 17:11-21 (2010)

Backx, FJ, et al. *Evaluation and opportunities in overtraining approaches.* Research Quarterly for Exercise and Sport 80-4 (2009): pp 756-64

Spaeth AM; Dinges DF; Goel N. *Effects of experimental sleep restriction on weight gain, caloric intake, and meal timing in healthy adults.* SLEEP 2013;36(7): pp 981-990

About the author

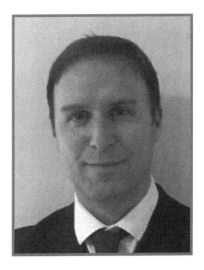

James Murray is the founder of Bellmate Systems and the Kinetic Fit programme. He has delivered personal training to professional athletes, celebrities and has spoken at nutrition and posture seminars for the NHS.

James is currently developing the new Kinetic Fit system and innovating and designing exciting new fitness products for the home and gym environments.

Visit *www.bellmatesystems.com* and claim your
Free One Month Access
to the complete Kinetic Fit System
Access Code: NDTDAD54

Made in the USA
Charleston, SC
10 November 2016